RADIOIMMUNOASSAY OF ANTIBODY
and its Clinical Applications

David Parratt
Department of Bacteriology,
Ninewells Teaching Hospital and Medical School,
Dundee, Scotland

Hamish McKenzie
Formerly Department of Bacteriology and Immunology,
Western Infirmary, Glasgow, Scotland

Klaus H. Nielsen
Animal Diseases Research Institute,
Nepean, Ontario, Canada

Present Address:
Department of Veterinary Pathology,
Texas A & M University,
College of Veterinary Medicine,
College Station, Texas 77843, USA

Susan J. Cobb
Department of Bacteriology and Immunology,
Western Infirmary, Glasgow, Scotland

A Wiley–Interscience Publication

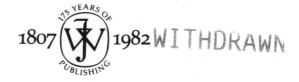

1807 1982 WITHDRAWN

JOHN WILEY & SONS
Chichester · New York · Brisbane · Toronto · Singapore

Library of Congress Cataloging in Publication Data:
Main entry under title:

Radioimmunoassay of antibody and its clinical applications.
  'A Wiley–Interscience publication.'
  Includes index.
  1. Radioimmunoassay. 2. Immunoglobulins—Analysis.
3. Chemistry, Clinical—Technique. 4. Biological
chemistry—Technique. I. Parratt, David.
QP519.9.R3R33   616.07'57   81-12939

ISBN 0 471 10061 7   AACR2

British Library Cataloguing in Publication Data:

Radioimmunoassay of antibody.
  1. Radioimmunoassay
  I. Parratt, D.
  616.07'56   RB46.5
ISBN 0 471 10061 7

Typeset by Preface Ltd., Salisbury, Wilts.
Printed at the Pitman Press Ltd., Bath, Avon.

269733

RADIOIMMUNOASSAY OF ANTIBODY
and its Clinical Applications

Dedication

*We dedicate this volume to our respective
spouses, whose forbearance has been considerable,
and at times 'beyond the call of duty'.*

Preface

This book is an attempt to draw together relevant information on the use of radioimmunoassay of antibody. We have frequently been asked by interested persons where they can find the relevant information about the method and who could teach them the 'tricks'. We taught as many as we could at the bench, but it was impossible to accommodate all, and we always had difficulty in referring them to published works. Our original answer, therefore, was to compile a set of working laboratory sheets, but in the process it became clear to us that there was more information than we had originally considered and that it was applicable to a wider audience than we had intended.

In compiling the volume we were torn between a simplistic, even dogmatic style, of benefit to the novice, and the more complex approach of reviewing the literature for the expert. We adopted a compromise in which most of the information is given simplistically, but where we felt that more detail was required, we have reviewed the available material in depth. Some chapters are therefore heavily referenced, others hardly at all, but in all instances we hope the reader will be provided with a starting point for further work.

Our critics would argue that radioimmunoassay of antibody is unnecessary, costly and dangerous. On the last two counts we discuss in the book counter arguments which we believe the reader will find compelling. As to necessity—we are all clinical microbiologists who believe that an immune response is a response and not just another immunological measurement. In short, our understanding is of a dynamic relationship between a host and a microorganism, or a host and an inert antigen, and we believe that to comprehend the interactions which are occurring in such a balance we require the most sensitive and flexible methods of assessment possible. For the study of humoral immunity this is undeniably radioimmunoassay of antibody or immune complexes. Nevertheless, it is only fair to the reader to say that we do not put diagnosis first. An understanding of the host/parasite/antigen interaction must come first, and diagnosis will then follow as a matter of course; in this we differ from many of our microbiological and immunological colleagues. We feel, though, that this approach is justified and that it has in part already been vindicated. Our colleagues are pleased if they can measure changes of antibody level over days or weeks, whereas we wish, and have achieved, analysis over hours.

Our critics would argue that to produce a book on radioimmunoassay of antibody is ill-timed when enzyme-linked (ELISA) assays are becoming popular. Our answer is that whilst ELISA may be useful for assays of 'antigen', there is little evidence that it is as good as radioimmunoassay for the measurement of antibody. Where the ELISA and radioimmunoassay for antibody measurement have been compared, there is no doubt that the latter method is more sensitive and accurate. Because we believe that a detailed understanding of antibody dynamics is essential we remain committed to the use of radioimmunoassay.

Nevertheless, the ELISA principle for measuring antibody is very similar to that of radioimmunoassay and we originally intended to discuss the former method in this book. It became clear that this was not possible for two reasons. Firstly, ELISA techniques have rarely been compared with radioimmunoassay so that a true picture of the differences has not yet emerged, though where there has been comparison in the measurement of antibody, radioimmunoassay has proved superior. The second reason is that where ELISA results have been reported, little information on the background of the assay has been given. Such important aspects as the assessment of antigen and antiglobulin excess, determination of 'labelling' density, substrate density, controls and standardization, have been almost totally ignored. To give an example, most reports on the use of ELISA for assay of antibody indicate that an absorbance reading above 0.2 is 'significant'. There is usually no definition of 'significance' in terms of what the antibody response means and no indication of how the standardization was achieved. The practice, in short, has been little better than that applied to 'conventional' assays of antibody such as the agglutination test or the complement fixation test. It is true that ELISA is more sensitive and easier than most of the conventional assays, but this is not the point. Any modern, sophisticated method of assay should improve our understanding of antibody responses and ELISA to date does not seem to us to have managed this.

Finally to the readership. The intended reader is someone who has no experience of radioimmunoassay, but has a need, either diagnostic or research, for improved analysis of humoral immune responses. We have attempted to include for such a person all the necessary information which is required to operate and adapt radioimmunoassay of antibody successfully. Nevertheless, we feel that a wider readership might find the text interesting, particularly those who are involved in serological analysis of any type. In this context, it is important to remember that clinicians are the ones who eventually have to interpret the results of serological tests. They should understand the principles, including new principles, which are used in the measurement. We have attempted in some parts of this book to incorporate a 'clinical' approach, notably in Chapters 1, 7 and 9, and we hope that practising clinicians will read and find useful the interpretation we give.

Our view then, is that radioimmunoassay of antibody is not just another method of detecting or measuring antibody which will aid diagnosis. It is a sophisticated technique which can, if properly used, provide the means by which immunological theory is applicable to an individual patient, with consequent improvement in his management. Whilst much of our text is basic, and deals with the methodology, we ask the reader to keep in mind this essential objective.

1981

David Parratt
Hamish McKenzie
Klaus H. Nielsen
Susan J. Cobb

Contents

Acknowledgements

We are indebted to many of our colleagues, who over the years have contributed ideas and technical assistance to the work contained in this book. In particular we would like to thank Dr W. J. Herbert for advice, and with his colleague Mr V. S. Mandranjan for the basic computer program. We appreciate also the help of Dr G. Boyd, whose clinical acumen and appraisal was so necessary to our studies of RIA of antibody. Special thanks are required to Mr P. F. H. Dawes who diligently reviewed the typescript, and to Miss V. Tait, Mrs V. Nolan, Miss W. Miller and Ms. Joan Graham who were the typists. Our thanks also to the Medical Illustration Department, and the Medical Physics Department, Ninewells Hospital. Furthermore, we are particularly indebted for the helpful advice and encouragement of Professors R. G. White and J. P. Duguid.

Finally, we would like to acknowledge the help and assistance provided by our publishers.

Chapter 1

General serological principles

INTRODUCTION

The measurement of antibody was one of the earliest adventures in immunology. At the time, the exercise was carried out by microbiologists who had little idea of the complexity of the substances they were studying, and whose goal was that of diagnosis of infectious disease, which at the time was a sore and oppressive ill. Nevertheless, the early workers discovered that antibody was formed against all things foreign, that it was specific and that it activated a serum factor (now called complement) and generally assisted in the removal of microorganisms from the body by phagocytic cells. The methods of assay of antibody which they developed were simple and applicable by most laboratories. In the main they consisted of agglutination tests where a serum was tested for its ability to clump a suspension of the microorganism of interest, or precipitation tests where an extract of the organism was used to 'precipitate' the antibody. Complement fixation tests were developed subsequently where the presence of an antibody was 'inferred' by its ability to block a second complement-activated reaction (usually the haemolytic effect on erythrocytes). All of these procedures have stayed with microbiology to the present. They have been variously adapted but not radically changed, and it is interesting that the immunologist has over the years adapted the same techniques to his, often sophisticated, purpose without considering whether a better alternative exists.

This book considers the use of radioimmunoassay (RIA) for the measurement of antibody. We shall discuss the available methodology, and the reasons why we believe it has advantages over the conventional procedures which have been carried down from earlier times. To be brief, the advantages of RIA are its sensitivity, accuracy and specificity. These are properties which can only be appreciated from an understanding of the methods in use, and from careful application of these to each problem which the diagnostician or scientist faces. One of the most important difficulties with which the user of RIA has to contend is that the method is so much more sophisticated than the conventional procedures he understands well. Consequently, the theory which has been useful to him in serological work with the conventional tests is not wholly applicable to RIA and a different approach to diagnosis and investigation is required when using this technique. For this reason we shall consider the basis, and the theoretical background for the use of RIA in this first chapter.

It is important when considering the use of any new method to decide whether it is needed, and for what reasons it is required. In many instances the considerations are essentially economic, but one should not decide solely on the latter criterion. An improvement in analysis, in terms of sensitivity and accuracy, should always be the aim.

In the assay of antibody an improvement of analysis is particularly relevant, and this can be illustrated by considering the background to such assays under the following heads.

DIAGNOSTIC USE OF RIA OF ANTIBODY

General principles

As indicated above, the diagnostic use of antibody assays is classically concerned with the identification of infective disease. The theory can be simply stated as follows. If an organism infects an individual it may produce disease and at the same time it will stimulate the individual's immune response to produce antibody which, if detected will *infer* the presence of the microbial agent. It is important to realise that the immune response is not confined to antibody, but it is usual to attempt measurement of the antibody response because this is technically easier to perform than, say, measurement of a cell-mediated response (T-cell response) to the same organism. The events which occur in the process of infection can be summarized in diagrammatic form (Fig. 1.1).

Diagnosis by this method is retrospective and is always by inference only. Detectable antibody does not appear until 7–14 days after the infection, and one has to rely on the appearance of the antibody as being indicative of the particular organism involved. It is possible in some instances that an increase of antibody may be due to a so-called 'heterophile' response, where the antibody formed during the infection cross-reacts with an antigen from another organism which is not causing the infection. A good example of this occurs in typhus. The organism producing the infection is one of the Rickettsial species, but the antibody which is measured is reactive with a bacterial (Proteus) species. By association we have learned that an antibody response to Proteus OX19 is typical in cases of typhus due to *Rickettsia prowazekii*. The point is that this is only by association and experience. A strict scientific interpretation would be that the patient had been infected by Proteus OX19. In the example given, the association is too well known to produce problems and indeed provides a useful diagnostic method, but it illustrates clearly that antibody, measured *after* the event, can only *infer* a diagnosis and can never *prove* it.

A second problem with serological diagnosis is that it depends upon survival

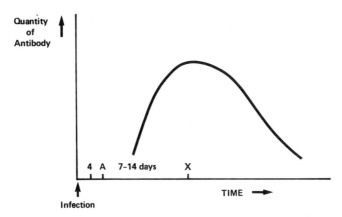

Figure 1.1. Diagrammatic representation of the antibody
response in infection. Note the late appearance of antibody

of the host for a period of time which will allow the diagnosis to be established. If (see Fig. 1.1) the patient succumbs at day 4, no detectable antibody has been produced and therefore no diagnosis is possible. Further, the only diagnosis possible by antibody analysis will be retrospective, and it can be argued that diagnosis in survivors is irrelevant. This is based on the assumption that the deployment of expensive tests to prove that a person has 'recovered' from a particular illness is a waste of resources. The arguments against this view are that (a) the recognition of the disease may have implications beyond the individual patient (e.g. typhoid) which affect the whole community and (b) the acute infection may lead to chronic disease which will require careful management (e.g. brucellosis—see Chapter 7). Although these are valid arguments, it is important to realise that the diagnosis has been based on inferences, and in practice it is often difficult to be certain that the serological diagnosis constitutes a basis for action, whether this be community action or action for the individual patient.

A justification for the use of delayed diagnosis is not, however, our primary aim, regardless of how valuable it may be. Our concern should be for diagnosis at the earliest stage of an infection so that the individual with the infection can be effectively treated and/or isolated. The patient who is likely to die is the one for whom diagnosis is most urgently required. It may be, and this is not always the case, that he will die *because* he fails to produce the antibody to neutralize the infecting organism. In such a case, conventional serological diagnosis will have little chance of success, but the alternative, that of isolation of the responsible microorganism, may be equally difficult. The isolation of microorganisms is often hampered by the difficulty of devising media and methods for obtaining a growth of the organism, and then by the technical problems of identifying the organism. For many bacteria and most viruses this is a formidable undertaking, and even when the organisms are isolated their significance is again inferred, and not *proved*, to be the cause of the patient's problems.

This is the basis of a fundamental principle which has been ignored in microbiology for a long time. The outcome in an individual patient depends not on whether he is infected with a particular organism (as inferred by isolation of that organism) or on whether he is responding to that organism (as inferred by serological diagnosis), but on *how well* he is responding to the particular organism. The latter question is rarely asked, and it is fundamental to any improvement of patient care. It does not abrogate responsibility of an epidemiological nature, but it focuses the investigation on the individual and his disease. Any diagnostic measure should, in brief, be capable of *proving* that an infection is present, and at the same time assessing the response of the patient to that infection. Inference is a poor substitute.

Advantages of RIA in assay of antibody

To achieve the above objective, however, requires a different approach to all diagnostic methods. We believe this can be achieved by proper assay of antibody and antigen/antibody complexes, but it is necessary first to consider the concepts on which conventional serological diagnosis are based.

Reference to Fig. 1.1 indicates that an increase of antibody infers a response to a particular infecting organism. If the patient is sampled at day X a high level of antibody is detected. This is taken by many to be proof that the organism has infected the patient. The rationale is that healthy patients will have little or no antibody, and can be easily distinguished from those with a high level. Indeed, in many instances like this, one is probably safe in assuming that such a large amount of antibody has been induced by an infection. However, it is not an infallible way of making the diagnosis because some individuals will produce large amounts of antibody in response to even minor contact with an organism. It may be, therefore, that the individual has not been infected, but only exposed and has produced a large response to the organism. This is rare but is important because it emphasizes again that a high level of antibody only *infers* the presence of infection. If the patient has symptoms at an appropriate time the corroborative evidence will suggest that infection has indeed occurred, but if the clinical picture is equivocal (as for example in a partially immune individual), the serological evidence will be insufficient to make the diagnosis.

The difficulties of attempting to diagnose an infection by a single, high level of antibody are well known to serologists, who have learnt from experience that the detection of a 'rising titre' is more satisfactory and accurate. Thus, referring to Fig. 1.1 again, if a sample were taken at A it would reveal no antibody, but a sample taken at X would have a high antibody level, and the difference between the two samples would indicate that antibody had been produced. A similar rationale is that once the infection is subsiding, antibody will disappear, so that a fall in level will be seen. It will be clear that to observe a rising titre will require about 7–10 days to elapse from the point of infection and to observe a fall may take considerably longer. In many instances, therefore, the information will be of only academic interest by the time it is obtained.

The concept of rising and falling titres has been developed with the use of conventional assays such as complement fixation, agglutination, neutralization and precipitation tests. Antibody has activity in two basic forms. The first is its ability to bind to its antigen, and this is a primary function. Its secondary, subsequent activity is its reaction in agglutination, complement fixation, neutralization and precipitation. Tests which use these activities do not measure antibody, or to be more precise they do not measure antibody–antigen binding, but rather they measure secondary *antibody activity*. In other words, when antigen binds to its antibody, some change occurs in the antibody which may be an important *biological* characteristic of the antibody. This change may allow the antibody to fix complement and then be detected by its complement-fixing properties. However, complement fixation is not an attribute of all antibodies. There are some immunoglobulins which cannot do this, e.g. human IgA, IgE and IgG_4 and others which are poor in this property (IgG_2). For these immunoglobulins complement fixation tests are useless, and it may be that the antibody response to an antigen in a patient is concentrated in one of these classes of immunoglobulin. Indeed, there is circumstantial evidence that this situation is common.

Virologists are particularly aware of the difficulty and note that neutralizing (but non-complement-fixing) antibody is often produced before complement-fixing antibody, and that the latter remains for longer periods after an infection (see Fig. 1.2). However, even when complement-fixing antibody is produced, its measurement is not always easy. The complement-fixing activity of any antibody is dependent on the antigen/antibody ratio, and this dependence is variable, as shown in Fig. 1.3. Most complement fixation tests allow for this problem by testing antibody and antigen at different concentrations, but it must be

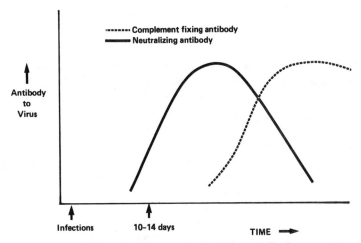

Figure 1.2. Diagrammatic representation of an antibody response to viral infection illustrating the relationship between neutralizing and complement-fixing antibody

6

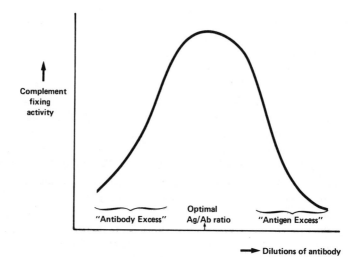

Figure 1.3. Diagrammatic representation of the complement fixation curve for constant amounts of antigen reacting with varying amounts of antibody

recognized that this makes the test cumbersome, and still open to some error. The error is recognized by most serologists, who will not regard the difference between two measurements as significant unless it is equal to or greater than 'four-fold' (i.e. at least 2 doubling dilutions). This is one of the reasons why it takes so long to make a serological diagnosis using such a conventional assay. One has to wait until the patient has increased his 'free' antibody by 400% before it is certain that the antibody level has passed the constraining limits of the assay which is being used to measure it. The proponents of such tests would argue that this is not a relevant question because the sensitivity of the system is high. Indeed, a properly established complement fixation test can measure antibody to levels of 0.1 μg (Humphrey and White 1970). It must be remembered that figures as low as these are only obtained for tests carried out under ideal circumstances (correct antigen/antibody ratios, complement concentrations and optimally sensitized red cells) and that such circumstances are unlikely to be possible for every sample in a 'routine' test on patients' sera. Thus the test is less than optimally sensitive, and is in addition inaccurate. These two features lead to the delay in detecting antibody, or a rising titre of antibody.

The problem of delay is not limited to complement fixation tests. With agglutination tests, for example, there is variability between antibodies in their ability to aggregate particles. This is used by some serologists who have reasoned that IgM is a better agglutinator than IgG, and therefore that agglutinating activity *infers* the presence of IgM antibody. This, as a generalization, is true, but there are many exceptions (e.g. non-agglutinating IgM, poor agglutinating IgM poor agglutinating IgG, good agglutinating IgG), and reliance on this technique leads to the same kind of inaccuracies and the same limitations as those described above for complement fixation tests.

Neutralization tests, particularly those used in the diagnosis of viral infections, are different. These tests, which are difficult to perform, depend on the ability of a patient's (serum) antibody to neutralize a standard inoculum of known virus. After allowing the serum and virus to react, the remaining infectivity is tested by seeding the mixture to a suitable layer of cultured mammalian cells. Several dilutions in duplicate or triplicate are required. After a few days, the presence of any live or non-neutralized virus can be detected by looking for death of cells in the culture. The importance of neutralization tests is that they show the *efficiency* of a patient's antibody in an activity which is important *in vivo* and experience has shown that such neutralizing antibody is usually protective. In contrast, complement-fixing antibody, which it could be argued would have a sufficiently destructive effect on microorganisms to be protective, cannot often be shown to provide protection. However, the complement fixation test is more convenient and complement-fixing antibody persists for longer than neutralizing antibody.

The problem with conventional precipitation assays is similar to that of complement fixation tests, because the precipitability may or may not be an attribute of a particular antibody, and the process of precipitation, if it is to occur, is dependent on optimal antigen/antibody ratios.

Therefore, dependence on the secondary biological activity of antibody for demonstrating and quantitating the antibody can produce delays and inaccuracy. The question which must be asked is whether antibody can be detected at an earlier stage by a more sensitive assay system.

The diagrammatic representation shown in Fig. 1.1 can be redrawn as shown in Fig. 1.4. This diagram includes the increase of population of the infecting microorganism and it can be seen that antibody becomes easily detectable only when it is produced in excess of the amount of antigen which is being generated by the microorganism. Prior to this, antibody is produced but is complexed with the antigens of the organism which may be cellular, insoluble or free and soluble substances. In molecular terms, any antibody in the serum which is bound to antigen (in antigen excess) has no free binding sites with which to attach to the antigen in an assay tube. Such a view is, however, simplistic because at any time in this early response some 'free' antibody will be available. This is because antibody–antigen reactions establish an *equilibrium* in which a varying proportion of antibody will remain free. Under conditions of excess antigen the amount of free antibody will be small, whilst in the reverse case of antibody excess large amounts of free antibody will be present in the serum. In the former case, conventional assays are usually incapable of detecting the small amount of available antibody and, as discussed above, one has to wait for antibody excess to be achieved. However, it is possible with very sensitive assays of antibody to detect this 'early' antibody and to define changes in the level of the antibody. Radioimmunoassay methods are invaluable for this type of work.

It will also be clear that an alternative means of diagnosis in the case given

8

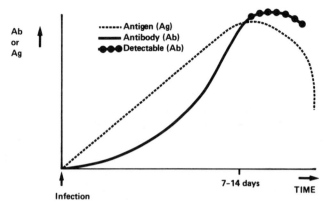

Figure 1.4. Diagram to indicate the relationship between microbial antigen and antibody to the antigen. The times are arbitrary but typical of many infections. Note the late appearance of *'free'* (i.e. detectable) antibody

above would be the detection of the antigen–antibody complexes, and here also radioimmunoassay is proving useful (see Chapter 7 for a detailed discussion).

Apart from the advantage of increased sensitivity, most radioimmunoassays have other assets which set them apart from conventional methods. Notable amongst these properties are (a) measurement of primary antigen–antibody binding as opposed to secondary antibody activity and (b) the ability to discriminate easily between different classes or subclasses of immunoglobulin.

The first of these has been discussed above, and is an advantage because, as indicated, reliance on the biological activity of the antibody may lead to problems where an antibody is incapable of performing a particular function. Thus IgM antibody may fail to agglutinate, or IgG antibody to precipitate. In both instances, however, the antibodies will bind to their antigens and detection of their binding will allow measurement. The second advantage is of considerable importance to the diagnostician. It is well known that after an antigenic stimulus, antibody is produced in a certain sequence. IgM antibody appears first and disappears early, is followed by IgG antibody, which persists for some time, and finally IgA is produced. This is shown diagrammatically in Fig. 1.5. The times are only approximate and there can be large departures from this generalized picture. Thus, IgM antibody may persist for months in some instances, although this would usually indicate persistent infection or administration of antigen. By analysing different classes of antibody it may be possible to infer the time of infection and therefore to establish the stage (early, middle or late) of the patient's infection. For example, in the diagnosis of brucellosis, the analysis is based on the concept that a direct agglutination test measures IgM antibody, whereas the indirect (Coombs) agglutination test measures IgG antibody. Whilst these simple techniques will be satisfactory for many test sera,

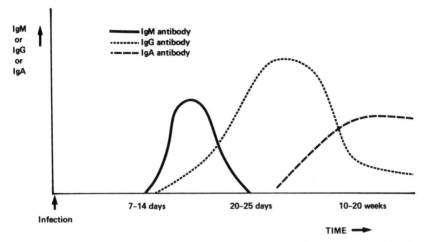

Figure 1.5. The sequence of antibody production of different immunoglobulin classes. The times given are arbitrary and provide only the overall pattern of a response to infection

they are not always reliable for reasons which have been discussed. A radio-immunoassay, on the other hand, using monospecific antiserum for the heavy chain of a particular immunoglobulin (e.g. IgM or IgG) will detect antibody only of the appropriate class and will not produce errors of interpretation or underestimations of the amount of antibody present. This is particularly valuable where the antibody is of a type which has no identifiable or distinct biological activity and which is therefore not detectable by conventional means. An example is IgA, which is sufficiently nondescript in a biological sense as to require immunochemical detection.

The same problem exists with the four subclasses of IgG in man. It is known that these subclasses have different properties, IgG_1 and IgG_3 being good for complement fixation, whilst IgG_2 is poor. IgG_4 is peculiar in that it sensitizes the individual and makes him susceptible to hypersensitivity reactions of a similar type to those induced by IgE (see Chapter 6). At present, analysis of the subclass response is a research area, but it is likely that within a short time such an analysis will be necessary for diagnostic purposes, and the only technique available will be radioimmunoassay or its equivalent. However, there are questions which are frequently raised against the use of radioimmunoassay: safety, ease of operation and cost. These are briefly discussed below.

Problems of RIA of antibody

Safety

There are many factors which influence the safety of radioimmunoassay, and it is difficult to summarize them concisely. Reference will be made throughout this book to various of these aspects, but here we shall aim to produce a general view.

Any radiation is dangerous, or potentially dangerous, and this should be clear to all who work with it. However, the dangers are greater where (a) the level of radiation is higher, (b) the radiation is particularly penetrating or (c) the radioactive isotope is liable to be trapped in the body. In the first instance, the amount of radiation handled in the laboratory will depend on the work load, and on the method of radiolabelling which is required for correct performance of the assay.

Some assays use very small amounts of isotope, as in the case of IgE PRIST assays (Chapter 6) where 10 μCi will be sufficient for 50 samples. The hazard here is low but is clearly related to the number of samples to be tested. In the average laboratory performing 200 such assays per month there is little problem, but an increase to 2000 samples per month may lead to difficulties. It may be unwise for a laboratory to convert all of its conventional serology to radioimmunoassay for this reason. The problem is greater where larger amounts of isotope are required for efficient performance of the assay.

Apart from these aspects, we must distinguish the two main stages of any assay procedure: 'labelling' of the reagents (usually antisera) where large amounts of radioisotope with consequent intense radiation are being handled, and the processing of the test sample where the levels are relatively low. The first procedure, if carried out by the investigator, must be carefully performed with the correct provisions for safety (see Chapter 3), but this step can sometimes be avoided by purchasing a reagent already labelled from a manufacturer. In the latter case, simple provisions for 'benchwork' are required provided, as indicated above, the necessary precautions for handling are observed (see Appendix).

As to the second point, that of the penetration of the radiation, most antibody radioimmunoassays use iodine-125, which has poor penetration except at short distances (up to 0.25 m). It is therefore easy, using lead shielding, to avoid any serious hazard. It must be noted that the use of iodine-131 may be more hazardous because this isotope emits radiation which is not so easily confined. In some ways it is fortunate that this isotope, with a shorter half-life, is not as popular as iodine-125, for reasons of convenience, and is infrequently used in antibody assay.

The third aspect is particularly important with isotopes of iodine, for these are concentrated in the thyroid gland where intense radiation in small areas may lead to necrosis of tissue or to the induction of tumours. Trapping of iodine isotopes in the thyroid will occur if the element is ingested or inhaled and it is therefore important when handling this material to maintain strict precautions regarding hand-washing, wearing of gloves, not smoking, etc., and at the same time to prevent aerosol formation (see Appendix). Trouble from this cause can, however, be effectively prevented by monitoring the amount of radioactivity in the thyroid gland, which can be done using a gamma counter (Mini-monitor) placed on the surface of the skin over the thyroid. The radioactivity, if recorded each week, will indicate those who are approaching maximum acceptable levels, and perhaps more important will determine whose technique is so poor as to allow this to happen.

Ease of operation

It is often thought that radioimmunoassays are difficult to perform. This is not so, and indeed most radioimmunoassays are simpler than alternative tests, particularly if the alternative is a complement fixation test. The qualification is that the assays are easy only if the correct equipment and facilities are available, and these in general are costly. Notes on the design of working areas and on the instrumentation required are given in the Appendix. However, most departments in western countries will have, or will have access to, the necessary facilities for antibody radioimmunoassay.

Cost

It is often thought that radioimmunoassays of antibody are more expensive than conventional procedures. If the capital cost of equipment and facilities is excluded, and costing is made on the basis of reagents and labour, they are usually equivalent to or cheaper than conventional assays. It is often said that enzyme-linked assays (ELISA) are cheaper than radioimmunoassays but the reagents and labour costs are little different between the two methods.

Finally, in any costing operation it is important to take into account two factors, (a) efficiency per cost and (b) applicability per cost. With the first of these, there is no doubt that radioimmunoassay is the most sensitive and accurate method of antibody quantitation yet developed, and this aspect will be expanded in later chapters. Thus for the cost it will give the best results, and in both research and diagnostic work this is an important consideration.

The second point, of applicability, is also important. A laboratory will often be equipped with apparatus, reagents and staff to carry out several different serological procedures all of which have the same ultimate objective, viz. measurement of antibody. Such policies, which are common, are illogical and expensive. It is better to use a single method which can be wholly or partially automated. Radioimmunoassay of antibody can be applied to the measurement of any antibody and is therefore a general procedure which could be adopted by the laboratory as a universally applicable method, provided that the amount of radioactivity used does not become too large.

RESEARCH APPLICATIONS OF RIA OF ANTIBODY

As mentioned in the previous section, radioimmunoassay is probably the most sensitive method of measuring antibody. Evidence can be found in studies of comparisons of methods, for example in the quantitation of antibody to herpes viruses (Friedman *et al.*, 1978), where a radioimmunoassay was considered to be 100 times more sensitive than either an enzyme-linked assay (ELISA) or immunofluorescence. Our experience is similar. For example, radioimmunoassays for the measurement of antibody to farmer's lung antigens can confidently quantitate levels down to 0.5 $\mu g/ml$, whereas immunofluorescence is inaccurate below levels of 30 $\mu g/ml$ (Parratt et al., 1975). By varying the conditions of assay (see Chapter 5), it is possible to make the radioimmunoassay even more sensitive.

The question is whether such sensitivity is useful. In many research projects it is, either because the amount of antibody to be measured is low, or because small changes in the level are of interest. The first of these situations may occur where the antibody co-exists with antigen (see above) so that 'free antibody' is in short supply. It is also important where the body is making only small amounts of the antibody, as in a quiescent 'maintenance' response, or where only small amounts of the antibody are normally produced, such as IgE antibody. Similarly, the amount of antibody in secretions is often low. In all of these instances it is important to remember that whereas the measurement of immunoglobulin may be easy, the measurement of specific antibody is not, and these situations and others are important areas for the researcher.

The second consideration, of change in antibody level, has already received some discussion above, in relation to diagnostic applications. However, it is often the purpose of the research to understand the *nature* of an immune response and, because this is dynamic, accurate monitoring of changes of antibody level is required over relatively short periods. For example, we have been interested in two aspects of antibody dynamics in human disease. The first is the removal of antibody from the circulating pool after challenge with a previously encountered antigen. This is an important question in extrinsic allergic alveolitis, where it is thought that the disease is caused by an Arthus-type hypersensitivity (i.e. antibody-mediated) to inhaled antigens. Theoretically, if the proposed mechanism is correct antibody should combine with the inhaled antigen in the lung and it should disappear from serum. Demonstration of a reduction in serum antibody levels during challenge provides good evidence that antibody is actually involved in the aetiology of the disease, and concurrently points the way to a better approach to diagnosis of the acute disease.

The data shown in Fig. 1.6 are from a study to demonstrate these events, and the antibody levels depicted were obtained using a radioimmunoassay for antibody to pigeon antigen (gamma-globulin) by a previously described method (Nielsen et al., 1974). The initial level of 15–16 $\mu g/ml$ of antibody, although significantly higher than normal (0–4 $\mu g/ml$), is below the level which would be detectable by the commonly used precipitin test, which only becomes positive above levels of 50–60 $\mu g/ml$. Here also the improved sensitivity of RIA is demonstrated. Further, the RIA clearly detects a fall in the level of antibody after antigen challenge, this being equivalent to a reduction of about 35%, which is followed after several days by a slow increase to levels slightly above the original 'resting' values. The decrease is rapid, and occurs soon after contact with the antigen. RIA of antibody is particularly useful for such studies of small,

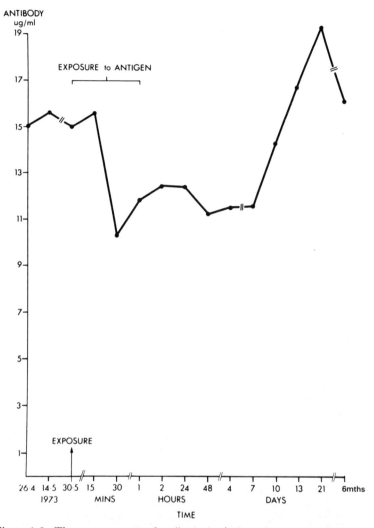

Figure 1.6. The measurement of antibody (μg/ml) to pigeon globulin in the serum of a patient with pigeon breeders' disease who had a trial exposure to the antigen. Note that the radioimmunoassay will satisfactorily measure changes over short and long intervals. (Reproduced by courtesy of Dr. G. Boyd, Royal Infirmary, Glasgow, and with permission of the *Scottish Medical Journal*)

rapid changes of antibody level, and the instance cited above is only one example where serial measurement of antibody under conditions of challenge can reveal useful information about the biology of the immune response.

The second aspect is the opposite of the above example and concerns the speed at which individuals respond to a new antigenic challenge. Fig. 1.7 contains information of antibody measurements to *C. albicans* in patients who had

14

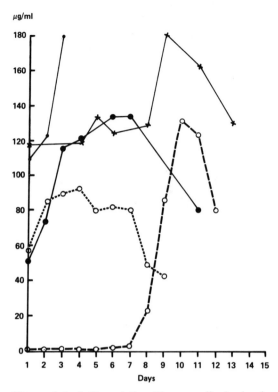

Figure 1.7. IgG anti-*C. albicans* antibody levels related to time (days) in patients undergoing intensive care. In all instances study began when the patients were admitted to intensive care and ended when they left. It is clear that there are considerable differences between different individuals in antibody response and it should be noted that most of the changes seen take place within 24-h intervals. The error of measurement by this RIA was ±5% and the range for healthy donors is 0–60 μg/ml.

been treated with broad-spectrum antibiotics. The effect of such drugs is to suppress the indigenous microflora of the intestinal tract and allow *C. albicans* to overgrow. This in turn produces a response to that organism, which varies in amount and speed in different individuals. It should be noted that antibody measurements here are being made over short periods of time and would be outside the scope of conventional assays for reasons which have been given above. Further, it is the delineation of the response in this sort of detail which is essential for the research worker who is attempting to find out why some such responses are successful and others are not.

We have restricted ourselves to simple examples in this section, for these are to serve only as illustrations and to indicate that where investigations of antibody reponses are required in detail the sensitivity and reproducibility of RIA is essential. It is worth noting that there is a paucity of information about antibody responses in humans, particularly in the early phase. This may be due to the fact that RIA and similar sensitive assays have been infrequently used.

GENERAL PRINCIPLES OF ASSAYS OF ANTIBODY

This section describes only the general features of these assays. Details of technique and precautions when carrying out the assays can be found in later chapters.

Direct Assays of antibody

The principle of these assays is that if antibody is allowed to react with its antigen it will bind to that antigen and thus become a target for an anti-immunoglobulin. The anti-immunoglobulin of a desired specificity is radiolabelled, and hence attachment of the radiolabel to the antigen will indicate that antibody is present in the test sample. Provided certain conditions are met (see Chapter 5 for details), the amount of radioactivity bound will reflect the amount of antibody present, and therefore measurement of the radioactivity leads to quantitation of the antibody. As with all radioimmunoassays, separation of bound and unbound radioactivity is required. In the direct assay of antibody, the antigen is always in the solid phase, either as a naturally occurring particle (cell, bacterium, etc.) or as an artificial product formed by attaching the antigen to a suitable solid-phase substance. Separation of bound and unbound material is therefore relatively easy and generally involves only washing and centrifugation. The procedure is outlined in diagrammatical form in Fig. 1.8. It is possible to use 'polyvalent' anti-immunoglobulin reagents which will react with all the different types of antibodies present, or to use mono-specific antisera against the major immunoglobulin classes, e.g. IgM, IgG, IgA. Thus the pattern of immunoglobulin response can be determined according to class, or even subclass, of the antibody.

Indirect or precipitation assays

In this type of assay the antigen and antibody mix and react in solution to form antigen–antibody complexes. The antigen component is usually radiolabelled and the principle of the method is therefore to separate the fraction containing antibody and to quantitate this by determining how much radioactivity it contains (Fig. 1.9). Larger amounts of radioactivity will indicate a greater degree of antigen–antibody binding and this can only have been achieved by a larger amount of antibody. The difficult part of the method is to separate bound and unbound radioactivity, that is, antibody–antigen complexes from remaining antigen. This is sometimes achieved by chemical or

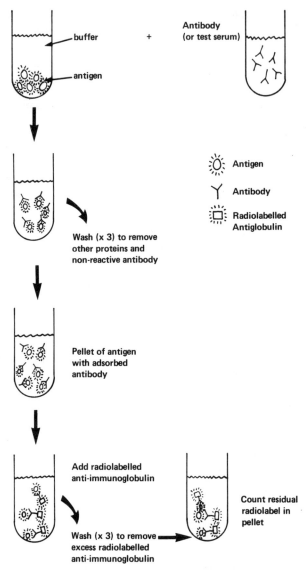

Figure 1.8. Diagram of the events occurring in a direct
assay of antibody

physical methods, or the use of a 'second antibody', an anti-immunoglobulin, to precipitate the original antibody. If the original antibody is complexed to radiolabelled antigen, radioactivity will be precipitated in the complex and measurement can then be performed. Detailed discussion of the means of precipitation and the method of calculating the amount of antibody in the sample is given in Chapter 4.

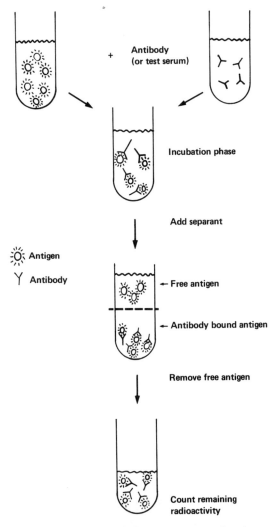

Figure 1.9. Diagram of the events occurring in a
competition assay of antibody

Throughout this first chapter, reference has been made to antigens and anti-bodies (particularly anti-immunoglobulins) as if they were easy to obtain. Indeed, sometimes these materials can be purchased or obtained from colleagues without too much difficulty, but more often the investigator will be required to prepare his own materials. In the next two chapters we discuss some of the methods employed for obtaining these reagents and discuss the problems which may be encountered. This discussion will begin with a consideration of the antigen preparation.

REFERENCES

Friedman, M. G., Haiken, H., Laventon-Kriss, S., Joffe, R., Goldstein, V., and Sarov, I. (1978). Detection of antibodies to varicella-zoster virus by radioimmunoassay and enzyme immunoassay techniques. *Med. Microbiol. Immunol.*, **166** (1–4), 177–186.

Humphrey, J. H., and White, R. G. (1970). *Immunology for Students of Medicine*. Blackwell Scientific Publications, Oxford and Edinburgh.

Nielsen, K. H., Parratt, D., Boyd, G., and White, R. G. (1974). Use of radiolabelled antiglobulin for quantitation of antibody to soluble antigens rendered particulate: Application to human sera from 'Pigeon fanciers' lung syndrome'. *Int. Arch. Allergy*, **47**, 339–350.

Parratt, D., Nielsen, K. H., Boyd, G., and White, R. G. (1975). The quantitation of antibody in farmers' lung syndrome using a radioimmunoassay: results of a clinical survey and comparison of three serological methods. *Clin. Exp. Immunol.*, **20**, 217–225.

Chapter 2

Antigens for radioimmunoassay of antibody

GENERAL ASPECTS

It is often stated that the strength of any radioimmunoassay is the antibody. This comment, undoubtedly true for hormone and other 'antigen' assays of competitive type, is founded on the principle that a good antibody will discriminate well. It could be argued similarly that for assays of antibody the antigen is just as important. As a general statement it is reasonable to suggest that without the correct antigen an assay of antibody will have little or no relevance. The selection of the antigen therefore requires some thought.

The first consideration in the case of assays for antibody to cells (e.g. micro-organisms or mammalian cells) is whether antibody to internal or external (cell wall or coat) antigens is to be measured.

The question is vexed, and different authorities will argue for one or other of these groups of antigens. It can be considered by looking at infections and responses to them. A forcible argument for the diagnostician is that if an organism invades and in the process is destroyed, its internal antigenic material will be released and will stimulate an antibody response. Alternatively, an organism which is not invading is unlikely to be destroyed and there will be no response to the internal antigens, only to the external or coat antigens of the organism. To measure antibody to the external antigens is said by the proponents of the 'internal antigen' principle, to indicate only exposure to the organism and to have no 'diagnostic' significance. It is true that antibody to 'internal antigen' is more frequently associated with disease than with simple exposure to antigen, but the concept that an antibody level must be 'diagnostic' is a limited one.

We have argued against this principle throughout this book (see Chapters 1 and 7). It is based on the notion that a level (in effect any level) of antibody must only be associated with disease in order to be useful to the diagnostician. Our argument is that a full and adequate description of any antibody *response* provides more information and offers an *understanding* of the processes which underlie the infection. Because of this, the detailed investigative approach can indicate ways of correcting an aberrant immune response and can provide more useful information for patient management.

Taking this alternative view, it is necessary to accept that the analysis of the antibody response must be undertaken from the view of the response as 'the organism sees it'. The 'picture' presented to the immune response will usually be that of an organism, multiplying in the body, and exhibiting its external or cell wall antigens, and the response to or increase of reactivity mounted against these antigens is the important measurement. Therefore, serial measurement of antibody to external or cell wall antigens is, arguably, the correct measurement for the diagnosis of infection.

It must be noted that this question is not resolved. Most investigators use one or other approach and argue their case along the lines above, but rarely apply both methods to the same problem.

CELL WALL PREPARATIONS

Whole cells

With many bacteria a suspension of organisms is all that is required for assay. One has to accept that the complexity of the antigens is great and that some will be better represented than others. Provided that preliminary estimations are carried out to ensure that antigen excess has been achieved (see Chapter 5), there should be little problem, although it is necessary to be certain that an excess of *all* antigens has been provided. This usually means that a large amount of suspension will be required for each assay tube. With bacteria this is usually possible because large amounts of the organism can be cultured. For viruses and a minority of bacteria, culture may be difficult and alternative methods are advisable (see below). Bacteria should generally be cultured on media which will not 'contaminate' the final suspension with proteins, especially those which cross-react with other reagents in the subsequent assay. In particular, blood or serum should not be present in culture media because these often harbour cross-reacting proteins. Generally, the best policy is to grow bacteria as a lawn on basic solid media. After suitable incubation the growth can be scraped off with a glass slide and collected and suspended in saline (0.15 M NaCl) or phosphate-buffered saline (PBS). The organisms should be killed by the gentlest method possible, in order to avoid disruption or distortion of their antigens. Heat (up to 65 °C for 30 min) or chemicals (e.g. sodium azide at a concentration of 0.5% or formaldehyde at a concentration of 0.4–1%) are frequently useful, but experimentation will be required to determine the best method for each organism.

After killing the organisms the suspension should be washed several times with PBS and made up to a final concentration of 5–50% (v/v). The concentration chosen will ultimately depend on the range of antibody levels to be measured, and will be determined by the need for antigen excess (see Chapter 5). However, a reasonable 'first choice' would be the use of a 10% suspension. If this is shown to be ineffective, a larger volume of suspension can be used or a new suspension of higher concentration can be made.

Some organisms prepared in this way will agglutinate. This is a problem for most radioimmunoassays because it makes efficient washing impossible. It is necessary, therefore, to disperse the organisms prior to testing. Dispersal can often be achieved by adding a small amount of protein (usually human albumin at a concentration of 0.1%) to the suspension, or by adding a detergent (e.g. Tween 20 or Triton X-100) at a concentration of 0.01% or EDTA (5–10 mM). Mild ultrasonication may also be useful, but must not disrupt the antigens of the cell. If these manoeuvres do not improve the quality of the suspension an alternative procedure, using a different solid-phase principle, should be adopted (see below).

Bacteria which will not grow on basic media and require an enriched medium can be spread on a layer of Cellophane resting on the surface of the medium. The organisms growing on the surface of the Cellophane can extract nutrients but they can be harvested cleanly and free of contamination by products from the medium.

The preparation of viruses for antibody assay is a formidable problem. These microorganisms grow only in tissue cultures (i.e. living cells) and the tissue cultures themselves require serum and other protein additives, all of which may be cross-reactive if they are present in the final antigen preparation. Producing a suspension of viral particles free of these materials may require considerable preliminary investigation. The first difficulty is to remove the virus particles from the cells. There are two basic means of doing this. The first is to rely on the 'natural' disruption of the cells which releases viruses into the supernatant fluid. In effect, one simply 'harvests' the supernatant culture fluid, replacing it with fresh medium and repeating the cycle several times. The pooled supernatants should contain the virus, which can be concentrated by ultracentrifugation (e.g. 10–20,000 g for 1 h). Contaminating proteins in the pellet of virus can be removed by repeated washing and centrifugation cycles. This inevitably is time consuming, but necessary.

The second method for harvesting virus is to disrupt the cells by ultrasonication, in which a mixture of virus, cell fragments and proteins is obtained. Removal of the virus cleanly from the mixture is difficult. The first stage is to deposit cell fragments and other large particles by centrifugation at $3000\,g$ for 10–30 mins, leaving the virus in the supernatant. The virus can then be sedimented as described above, although it must be remembered that any remaining cell fragments of the same size as the virus will also be deposited. Several cycles of centrifugation under different conditions may be necessary and the actual preparative conditions for each antigen must be pre-determined by experiment. It is likely, even so, that the virus preparation will remain contaminated, and the contamination may be greater than that produced by the first method of preparation. However, the yield of virus particles is likely to be higher after induced disruption of the cells, and may compensate for the deficiencies of the separation.

It will be clear from the above that centrifugation of viral particles is time consuming and because an essential part of the basic direct RIA of antibody involves several centrifugation steps after thorough washing of the antigen-bearing particle (see Chapter 5), simple suspensions of viruses prepared in this way are rarely suitable for assay. Attachment of the virus to a solid-phase particle or substrate is generally better and the available materials and methods for this are discussed below.

Antigenic cross-reaction

Another topic to be considered when preparing any microorganism as an antigen for assay is that of cross-reaction. Most organisms contain tens or hundreds of antigens, and inevitably some of these antigens will be present in other microorganisms (i.e. common rather than specific antigens). This kind of cross-reaction is well known amongst bacteria of the Enterobacteriaceae class. It could be argued that if the antigens contained in a suspension of microorganisms cross-react with antigens from other species of microorganism, diagnosis by assay of antibody is impossible. By conventional theories this is true, because a diagnostic 'titre' of antibody to one and only one organism, is required for diagnosis. It is imperative in this view to have available a specific (i.e. to the one organism) antigen and to look for antibody to that antigen. Such a view, despite its practical value in the past, is now naive. The fact is that an individual who is infected will respond to all *available* antigens, whether they are cross-reactive or not, and if serology is to mean anything it should analyse the complexity of the response and predict the outcome. Cross-reactive antigens are just as important as the specific ones, perhaps more so, because an individual may respond quickly to a cross-reacting antigen which he has experienced before. The choice for the investigator is to decide whether he wishes to make a simple diagnosis by using a single, specific antigen or whether he wishes to use serology to analyse the complexity of immune responses towards a wider interpretation of hose–parasite or host–antigen interactions. If the latter way is chosen, cross-reacting antigens become irrelevant and it is a major tenet of this book, emphasized in Chapter 1, that the wider approach to serology can be successful if sensitive methods such as RIA are used.

The discussion above has considered the use of preparations of whole cells or cell wall fragments. However, the internal products of the organism, as already indicated, may be important antigens against which an infected host will respond. The internal components are soluble proteins, often enzymes, and must be attached to a suitable solid phase before they can be used in RIA. The sections below consider the ways in which this can be achieved. Here, an outline is given of methods for disruption of the microorganisms.

INTERNAL ANTIGENS

Preparation with hypotonic solutions

The simplest of all hypotonic materials is, of course, distilled water. Some microorganisms, such as the protozoan trypanosomes and spirochaetes such as

Treponema pallidum, will lyse in distilled water. Many bacteria, particularly gram-negative forms, will be disrupted although not completely, but most gram-positive bacteria will resist this treatment. Yeasts and fungi are very resistant. The advantages of this method are that it is simple and the released antigens are not seriously damaged. The supernatant fluid, after several hours in contact with the organism, is dialysed against a physiological buffer such as PBS (pH 7.2) before the antigens are attached to a solid phase. It may be necessary to change the pH again for the latter process if, for example, attachment to plastic is chosen (pH 9.2). This is preferably done slowly, in two steps, to allow the proteins to regain their structure before being subjected to another non-physiological buffer. Although the method is simple, it must be added that the yield of antigen is not usually as high as it might be using alternative techniques.

Hypotonic buffers may be used as an alternative to distilled water, but it will be clear that the yield with these is often poor, even though antigen distortion does not usually occur.

Preparation by freeze-drying

This is another simple and readily available method. Freeze-drying is a standard procedure for preserving microorganisms in a recoverable state for long periods. However, only a small percentage of the microorganisms survive the process. Those which perish disintegrate when the culture is reconstituted, and in so doing release their internal antigens into the supernatant fluid used for reconstitution. The yield of antigen obtained in this way is often high and the method is particularly useful for 'tougher' gram-positive bacteria.

Preparation by freezing and thawing

The same result as that obtained with freeze-drying can be achieved by subjecting a suspension of microorganisms to repeated cycles of freezing and thawing. The advantage is that expensive freeze-drying equipment is not essential, and this process can be performed in the freezing compartment of an ordinary refrigerator, although preferably in a deep-freezer at $-20\,^{\circ}$C. The disadvantage is that several (up to ten) cycles of freezing and thawing are necessary. After completing the procedure the suspension of microorganisms should be examined microscopically to ensure that disruption has occurred, and the product should then be centrifuged ($3000\,g$ for 10–30 min) to remove cell wall debris. A high yield of antigen can be obtained in this way. If adequate disintegration is not achieved, the suspension can be further treated by ultrasonication (see below). There is, however, a danger that some of the antigens released will be distorted by freeze-thawing or ultrasonication.

Preparation by ultrasonication

Any cells, whether microorganismal or mammalian, can be disrupted by ultrasonication. It should be noted, though, that the energy directed on the cells by this method is considerable and consequently protein disintegration or damage is likely to occur unless care is taken to establish optimum conditions. The principle is that a beam of ultrasonic waves is directed into a suspension of the organism and when the beam hits the organisms the energy is absorbed by the cells, resulting in damage. Inevitably, heat is generated and in the immediate zone of impact the temperatures are extremely high. In the process any released antigens are heated and may be denatured. It is usual to hold the suspension in an ice-bath whilst the ultrasonic bombardment proceeds, but this is simply to prevent the suspension from boiling, and has little influence on the high temperatures achieved at the point of impact of the energy waves. If this method has to be used it is essential to monitor the antigen carefully by testing its performance against an antibody-containing standard antiserum. Also, it is preferable to use short periods of ultrasonication frequently rather than a single period of heavy radiation (e.g. ten cycles of 30 s rather than one 5-min exposure). The intervals between each 'burst' of radiation treatment should be at least 30 min. At the end of the procedure, the preparation should be examined for the absence of whole microorganisms (by microscopy) and for the presence of intact antigens (by assay against a 'standard' antiserum).

Culture solutes

Many of the 'internal' antigens of bacteria, fungi and protozoa are enzymes, and are excreted into the environment. Because these enzymes are complex proteins they are antigenic and in an infected host they will produce an antibody response. Indeed, some investigators believe that the only relevant antigens are enzymes (Walbaum et al., 1969) and that if the host has not responded to these, there is no serological indication of disease. This is a contentious and unresolved question, which cannot be discussed here for reasons of space, but a mention of the methods for obtaining these enzymes is necessary. The 'traditional' method is to disrupt the microorganism by one or more of the techniques described above, and to 'purify' the product by chromatography, or affinity chromatography, using immunochemical techniques for monitoring. This type of work, however, is complex and time consuming.

A simpler way of obtaining enzyme antigens is to disrupt the medium on which the organisms have been growing, for this will contain high concentrations of the enzymes. With bacterial cultures, the culture medium is scraped clean of the bacteria and then disrupted by freezing and thawing. This releases much of the water from the agar and any enzymes will be removed with the water. Collection of the fluid from several plates and concentration after centrifugation to remove cell debris will usually produce a potent mixture of enzyme antigens. Further processing of these should be as indicated below.

There are other methods for disruption of microorganisms, such as phage lysis, enzyme digestion and antibiotic treatment, which could be discussed, but these have not yet come into common use. No doubt these and other methods will be employed in the future. It is necessary for each investigator to consider the nature of antigen required for his assay and to adopt or adapt one or more of the available methods.

Having produced, by any of these methods, a soluble antigen, the next problem is how to prepare it for radioimmunoassay. Some of the available techniques are discussed below.

SOLUBLE ANTIGENS IN RIA

General Aspects

Particulate antigens such as microorganisms or erythrocytes can be easily separated from other components in a radioimmunoassay mixture by centrifugation, and the preparation of these antigens has been described above. However, to measure antibody to a soluble antigen, a method of linking the antigen to a solid support must be found if the convenience of a solid-phase assay is to be exploited. Historically, this problem was solved in conventional serology by adsorbing soluble antigens to the surface of erythrocytes which had been treated with tannic acid (Boyden, 1951). Such antigen-linked red cells have been widely used in agglutination assays and other conventional methods, but have two main disadvantages:

1. The antibody assay must be performed under mild reaction conditions in order to avoid haemolysis of the cells.
2. Antibodies to 'heterophile antigens' on the erythrocytes surface are fairly common, and may produce 'false positive' results.

Thus attempts have been made to find inert solid supports which will not participate in antigen–antibody interactions, and which will remain stable under the operating conditions of the assay. These inert solid supports are particularly important for radioimmunoassay of antibody.

Adsorption to plastic supports

In 1956, polystyrene latex particles were introduced as a solid-phase adsorbent for rabbit globulin, and used in agglutination tests for rheumatoid factor (Singer and Plotz, 1956). Similar particles have subsequently been used by Klinman and Taylor (1969) for adsorbtion of protein-like haptens in a solid-phase antibody radioimmunoassay. Further, Catt and Tregear (1967) found that antibody could be adsorbed to the surface of polypropylene or polystyrene tubes, and these workers used the immobilized antibody for a competitive assay of radiolabelled antigen. The immobilization of protein antigens on polymeric plastics has since been widely used in RIA of antibody, with either tubes, plates or spherical particles as the solid support. The principle is the same for each of these, and the choice depends largely on practical considerations. For example, latex particles have to be dispensed in suspension and centrifuged during the washing procedures, with the possibility that some of the material may be lost during washing. In contrast, this is unlikely to occur with plates or tubes, which require only that the wash buffer be poured on and off. However, plates do present a problem when it comes to counting the radioactivity in individual wells at the completion of the assay. The wells must be separated in some way, which is usually achieved by dismemberment with a heated wire.

With all of these methods, the optimum conditions for adsorption of an antigen to a plastic support should be determined for each assay system. The basic pattern is simple. A solution of antigen at a neutral or alkaline pH is left in contact with the plate/tube/particles, and allowed to incubate overnight at 37 or 4 °C. The solid phase is then washed in assay buffer and re-incubated with an excess of a protein which is unrelated to the antigen [usually 0.5% (w/v) bovine serum albumin]. This step ensures that any remaining protein binding sites on the plastic support are 'occupied', and after further washing in assay buffer the solid-phase antigen is ready for use. Among the variables which may be worth optimizing are the concentration of antigen, the pH of binding, the incubation temperature and the length of incubation.

Prat and Comoglio (1976) linked increasing concentrations of a soluble membrane antigen to plastic plates and studied the binding of antibody by the immobilized antigen. They found that with increasing antigen concentration more antibody was bound until a maximum was reached. Above this maximum, higher antigen concentrations produced a decrease in the amount of antibody bound. They suggested that at very high antigen concentrations there is increased dissociation of antigen from the solid support, which results in less efficient antibody binding, although an alternative explanation is that the increased concentration of antigen molecules on the plastic surface caused steric hindrance and limited the access of antibody molecules to the 'hidden' antigen. Preliminary experimentation to find the best antigen concentration for binding is therefore probably essential.

Variations of the incubation conditions by different researchers are considerable, although this may be influenced by the nature of the antigen and its ability to resist denaturation rather than by the efficiency of the binding procedure. Catt and Tregear (1967) adsorbed antibody to plastic tubes at pH 9–10, whereas Hay et al. (1975) adsorbed rabbit IgG to tubes at neutral pH. Hay et al. incubated for 1 h at 37 °C, and then overnight at 4 °C, whereas Clague et al. (1979) bound bovine collagen to plastic tubes with only an overnight incubation at 4 °C, ostensibly to minimize denaturation of the collagen.

In addition to purified protein antigens, plastic adsorbents have been used for more complex antigen mixtures, and even for cells. Lange et al. (1976) have used the technique to immobilize DNA for an assay of anti-DNA antibody in sera from patients with connective tissue disease. Nowinski et al. (1979) adsorbed a murine leukaemia virus to plastic plates by overnight incubation at 37 °C in PBS, and Friedman et al. (1979) successfully immobilized a sonicate of human fibroblasts which had been infected with varicella zoster virus.

However, when using cells or fragments of cells a 'fixative' may be helpful. Stocker and Heusser (1979) attached leucocytes and erythrocytes to plates by first centrifuging a layer of cells to the bottom of each well, and then fixing them by immersion in 0.25% glutaraldehyde in PBS at 4 °C for 1 h. Huang et *al.* (1975) similarly immobilized tumour cells on plastic plates using 10% neutralized formalin.

The use of plastic adsorbents is not limited to soluble antigens, and can be usefully extended to intact cells. In this way, the technique of solid-phase radioimmunoassay can be applied to particulate antigens which are too small to be conveniently centrifuged in the washing procedures necessary during the RIA. This is particularly useful with viral particles, prepared by the methods described above, or with small fragments of some larger microorganisms such as bacteria. Indeed, some whole bacteria (e.g. *Brucella*) produce a very fine suspension which is difficult to centrifuge and it may be that these organisms are better suited to assays in which they are bound to a solid-phase support. However, attachment of these particles to the support will usually require treatment with 0.25% glutaraldehyde.

It is our view that if antigen attachment to a platic/polystyrene support is possible, it should be used. The advantage is that washing during the assay, counting and storage of the material is simpler, and simplicity leads to higher accuracy. A problem which some investigators have encountered is non-specific attachment of other (serum) proteins to the plastic support during the assay. This may cause either underestimation or overestimation of the test sample, and unless care is taken this difficulty may not be recognized. However, if the assay includes a 'blank' (i.e. saline) control, it will become apparent for this control will record a higher activity than a 'normal serum' control, which is known to have no antibody to the antigen (see Chapter 5). Having recognized the problem it is preferable to avoid it and this can be achived by saturating any excess protein-binding sites, after linking the specific antigen to the adsorbent, with a buffer containing a low [i.e. 0.5% (w/v)] concentration of human or bovine serum albumen.

An alternative to the use of plastic adsorbents is to use a more 'active' support such as one of the cyanogen bromide-activated materials which are described below.

Adsorption to cyanogen bromide-activated materials

The use of cross-linked dextrans such as Sephadex® or Sepharose® as a solid support matrix for soluble antigens became possible when Axen *et al.* (1967) described the cyanogen bromide method of covalent linking of proteins to these materials. After cyanogen bromide activation, Sephadex® and Sepharose® will react with any primary amino group to form a *stable* dextran–antigen conjugate. The procedure will also work with cellulose discs (see Chapter 6).

It is possible to purchase Sephadex® or Sepharose® which is cyanogen bromide activated, and for most laboratories this is undeniably the best approach to the use of these materials. However, cyanogen bromide activation of the basic materials (which is cheaper) by the investigator is simple, provided that precautions are taken as cyanogen bromide is highly poisonous and volatile. The basic method is as follows.

Sephadex® G-10 or Sepharose® is mixed with cyanogen bromide (25 mg/ml) and the pH is maintained at 10.5 for 2 min using 2 M NaoH. The pH must be frequently checked by 'spotting' small amounts of the reaction mixture on to pH paper of an appropriate range, and the alkali added quickly as the mixture becomes acidic. After holding the mixture for 2 min under alkaline conditions it is transferred to a filter (e.g. fitted to a Buchner flask under vacuum) and washed thoroughly with distilled water. Thereafter the material is dried by successive washes with 50, 75 and 100% (v/v) acetone in distilled water. The whole operation must be carried out in an efficient fume cupboard and gloves, protective goggles and a gown should be worn.

Having obtained the cyanogen bromide-activated material, the next step is linkage of the antigen. This is accomplished by incubating the antigen with the activated support for 1–4 h at room temperature at an alkaline pH (8.5). The support is subsequently washed in an alkaline buffer to remove unbound antigen and excess binding sites are 'saturated' with 0.1 M ethanolamine (in 0.1 M bicarbonate) for 2 h. The material is then washed once with 0.2 M acetate buffer (pH 4.0), the same buffer is replaced and the mixture is allowed to stand at 4 °C for 1 h before final washing and resuspension in PBS (pH 7.2).

The alkaline conditions for linking are usually achieved with 0.1 M bicarbonate buffer. We have found recently that the linkage of antigen is often better if it is mixed with the solid support for 4–5 days at 4 °C with mechanical agitation.

If cyanogen bromide-activated Sepharose® is purchased, the manufacturers will supply full details of the linkage procedure which they consider the best.

It is worth noting that any 'antigen' molecule which possesses a primary amino group will bind to the activated material, and therefore the method is applicable when non-protein antigens are being investigated, provided of course that these possess an amino group (e.g. antibiotics). This has been used by us to measure antibody to ampicillin in infectious mononucleosis (McKenzie et al., 1976).

However, the versatility of linkage is not restricted to this sort of instance. There is available a range of substitute Sepharose-like products which permit antigens to be bound by other functional units, including hydroxyl (useful for carbohydrates), thiol and carboxyl groups. With these substances, virtually any antigen can be linked to a Sepharose-type matrix. Guidance on the appropriate type of Sepharose® for any particular antigen can be obtained from the manufacturer's literature (Pharmacia Fine Chemicals Ltd.).

Despite the simplicity of attaching antigens to these activated supports, problems in the subsequent assay can arise. Notably, small antigens such as drugs or low molecular weight hormones may be bound so tightly to the matrix that antibody molecules (in the test serum) cannot attach to them. If this problem arises or is suspected, a 'spacer' molecule such as gelatin or a synthetic amino acid sequence should be attacked to the activated material, and the antigen of interest attached to this by mild treatment with glutaraldehyde (0.25%).

The cyanogen bromide method can also be used to activate filter-paper discs (cellulose or paper) in the same way as for Sepharose.® The activated disc, once 'tagged' with antigen, is a useful reagent for RIA for antibody because it is easily processed. This type of solid-phase antigen is used in the PRIST and RAST assays discussed in Chapter 6.

Although the methods of attachment of antigen to a solid phase, discussed above, are the commonly used ones and are convenient, they are not exclusive. We have, for example, resorted to a different technique for the attachment of pigeon globulin to a solid phase (Nielsen *et al.*, 1974). Briefly, we were interested in quantitating human antibody to pigeon globulin, which is an important antigen in pigeon breeders' disease (Chapter 1). Pigeons were therefore immunized with sheep red cells, and the antibody (i.e. globulin) which they produced was reacted with sheep erythrocytes. This produced sheep red cells coated with pigeon gamma-globulin, and this was the antigen for assay of human antibody (to pigeon globulin). Subsequently, we have used pigeon globulin attached to cyanogen bromide-activated Sepharose® with similar results, but the original method is mentioned to indicate that each investigator should be able, with a little ingenuity, to assay any antibody by a solid-phase method.

Finally, it must be noted that the ultimate choice of a solid substrate may not depend wholly on the antigen-binding properties of the latter, but on the availability of automation. An RIA of antibody, as will become apparent later, has its strength in its ability to measure small changes of antibody over short periods of time. It is to be expected, therefore, that these assays will have to handle multiple samples, and to deal with them quickly. In order to achieve efficiency in the assay, automation is clearly advisable, if not essential. The automation of assays using Sepharose® is difficult, whereas with polystyrene beads or microtitre plates it is simpler (the beads are undoubtedly easier to use).

We end this chapter with an example (see Fig. 2.1). It shows that the method of antigen preparation can be varied, without disrupting the performance of the assay, and indicates that the final test of any antigen is a practical one in the assay itself.

In this example, antigens from *Trypanosoma brucei brucei* were attached to Sepharose and used as a substrate for an assay of human IgG antibody. The trypanosomes were grown in mice and rats and after several days blood from the infected animals was collected and processed. The blood from the mice and the rats was separately processed by ion-exchange chromatogrpahy to concentrate the organisms. These were gently sonicated, and the resulting cell-free supernatant was bound to Sepharose® by the standard procedure (see above). The antigen derived from rats was compared with that from mice, using a single 'standard' serum which was known to have a high antibody level to the organisms. The standard serum was used at several dilutions.

It can be seen that the binding of antiglobulin, and therefore antitrypanosome antibody, was almost the same for each antigen, and that the regression line for each was the same. There was no 'plateau' effect even at high concentrations of antibody. This type of experiment indicates that antigens prepared in different ways should perform satisfactorily, provided that antigen

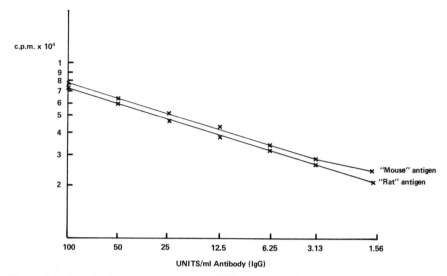

Figure 2.1. Results from an experiment which compared Sepharose–trypanosome antigens for reactivity with human antibody to the organisms. In one instance the trypanosomes were harvested from mice and in the other from rats (see text for details)

and antiglobulin excesses are achieved, and full technical precautions are taken (see Chapter 5).

Having selected a method of antigen preparation, the production of a discrimatory antibody (e.g. an antiglobulin) must be considered.

REFERENCES

Axen, R., Porath, J., and Ernback, S. (1967). Chemical coupling of peptides and proteins to polysaccharides by means of cyanogen bromides. *Nature (Lond.)*, **214**, 1302.

Boyden, S. U. (1951). The adsorption of protein on erythrocytes treated with tannic acid and subsequent haemagglutination by anti-protein sera. *J. Exp. Med.*, **93**, 107–120.

Catt, K., and Tregear, G. W. (1967). Solid-phase radioimmunoassay in antibody coated tubes. *Science*, **158**, 1570–1572.

Clague, R. B., Brown, R. A., Weiss, J. B., and Holst, P. J. (1979). Solid phase radioimmunoassay for the detection of antibodies to collagen. *J. Immunol. Meth.*, **27**, 31–41.

Friedman, M. G., Leventon-Kriss, S., and Sarov, I. (1979). Sensitive solid-phase radioimmunoassay for detection of human immunoglobulin G antibodies to Varicella zoster virus. *J. Clin. Microbiol.* **9** (1), 1–10.

Hay, F. C., Nineham, L. J., and Roitt, I. M. (1975). Routine assay for detection of IgG and IgM anti-globulins in sero-negative and sero-positive rheumatoid arthritis. *Br. Med. J.*, **3**, 203–204.

Huang, J. C.-C., Berczi, I., Froese, G., Tsay, H. M., and Sehan, A. H. (1975). A micro-radioimmunoassay for antibodies to tumour-associated antigens. *J. Nat. Cancer Inst.*, **55**, 879–866.

Klinman, N. R., and Taylor, R. B. (1969). General methods for the study of cells and serum during the immune response: the response to dinitrophenyl in mice. *Clin. Exp. Immunol.*, **4**, 473–487.

Lange, A., Roitt, I. M., and Doniach, P. (1976). A double antibody solid phase assay for DNA auto antibodies for clinical use. *Clin. Exp. Immunol.*, **25**, 191–198.

McKenzie, H., Parratt, D., and White, R. G. (1976). IgM and IgG antibody to ampicillin in patients with infectious mononucleosis. *Clin. Exp. Immunol.*, **26**, 214–221.

Nielsen, K. H., Parratt, D., Boyd, G., and White, R. G. (1974). Use of radiolabelled antiglobulin for quantitation of antibody to soluble antigens, rendered particulate. *Int. Arch. Allergy*, **47**, 339–350.

Nowinski, R. C., Lostrom, M. E., Tam, M. R., Stone, M. R., and Burnette, W. N. (1979). The isolation of hybrid cell lines producing monoclonal antibodies against the P15 (E) protein of ecotrophic murine leukaemia viruses. *Virology*, **93**, 111–126.

Prat, M., and Comoglio, P. M. (1976). A solid state competitive binding radioimmunoassay for measurement of antigens solubilised from membranes. *J. Immunol. Meth.*, **9**, 267–272.

Singer, J. M., and Plotz, C. M. (1956). The latex fixation test: 1. Application to the serologic diagnosis of rheumatoid arthritis. *Am. J. Med.*, **21**, 888–892.

Stocker, J. W., and Heusser, C. H. (1979). Method for binding cells to plastic: application to a solid phase radioimmunoassay for cell surface antigen. *J. Immunol. Meth.*, **26**, 87–95.

Walbaum, S., Biguet, J., and Tram Van Ky, P. (1969). Structure antigenique de *Thermopolyspora polyspora*. Repercussions practiques sur le diagnostic du 'poumon du fermier'. *Ann. Inst. Pasteur*, **117**, 673–693.

Chapter 3

Preparation of antisera and radiolabelling

PREPARATION OF ANTISERUM

General comments

The strength of any radioimmunoassay, in terms of its specificity and sensitivity, depends on the properties of the antiserum. In the context of assay of antibody, it follows that when IgG antibody is being measured, the antiserum (that is, anti-IgG) must measure this immunoglobulin only. Similarly, when IgM antibody is being measured the antiserum must be specific anti-IgM. The use of anti-whole immunoglobulins for the assessment of antibody is not in general satisfactory, because it is difficult to attain high activity against each Ig class in the same antiserum. It can be done by pooling different monospecific antisera in appropriate proportions, but this may be difficult to achieve. In general, a high degree of specificity is preferable and the anti-immunoglobulin should be of sufficient calibre to discriminate between very small amounts of antibody and none at all, and at the same time very high levels of antibody. For these reasons the antiserum to be used in the assay must be carefully selected.

Commercially prepared antisera are usually not satisfactory for radioimmunoassay of antibody, probably because they are not developed for this purpose but for the more general purpose of producing precipitin reactions for a different type of test. A notable exception is the anti-IgE antibody used in the RAST and PRIST systems, where the antiserum has been developed to a high degree by affinity chromatography, and where discrimination is good. However, this topic will be dealt with elsewhere (see Chapter 6).

In general, therefore, the investigator will be required to prepare his own antiserum, and this section deals with some of the methods and procedures which we have found to be valuable in producing our antisera. We do not presume that our methods are exclusive and the description given is only to provide a start for inexperienced workers and perhaps an indication of alternatives for those who have more experience of these matters.

32

There are two extremes which can be followed when preparing an antiserum. The first is to highly purify the immunogen, in this instance an immunoglobulin. This may take time, and the methods by which purification of immunoglobulin and anti-immunoglobulin can be achieved will be discussed below. If a purified immunogen is prepared and used to immunize an animal, an antiserum will be produced which is mainly reactive with the immunizing substance and will require only minimal absorption. It must be noted however, that absorption of all anti-immunoglobulins (including those prepared with purified immunoglobulins) is essential to remove activity against determinants common to all the immunoglobulins, such as the light chain determinants. Further, many animals will produce antibodies against commonly occurring microorganisms and these antibodies will be present in the prepared antiserum. It may be that when assays are being carried out for antibody against commonly occurring microorganisms the inherent or natural antibody present in the antiserum will interfere with the proper performance of the test, and lower its sensitivity. For these reasons absorption of such unwanted (specific but unwanted, not non-specific) activity is necessary. It should be noted that if the Fc portions of the immunoglobulin molecule are prepared and used as an immunogen, the resulting antiserum will be monospecific and requires no absorption of light chain activity, although antibody to common organisms will still need to be absorbed.

The second approach when preparing an antiserum is to use a fairly crude preparation of the immunogen and accept that the antiserum produced by the donor animal will be of wide specificity and will require absorption. In terms of time saved or time spent, both of these approaches are approximately equal. In other words, one either spends time preparing an immunogen and less time absorbing for specificity of the final product, or very little time preparing the antiserum and a lot of time absorbing for specificity and checking that specificity.

Our approach has been somewhere between the two extremes. Thus, in the preparation of an anti-IgG, we would take some steps to purify IgG by simple means (sodium or ammonium sulphate precipitation followed by QAE 50 chromatography; see below), and immunize with this preparation, accepting that the antiserum will require absorption with light chains or with IgG-deficient normal serum, and possibly with a range of microorganisms. It seems to us justified to follow this middle course because the best test of any antiserum is in the performance of the assay itself, and with obvious exceptions it is sometimes possible to achieve satisfactory results with antisera which are not prepared in the most exacting fashion. In other words, there are some benefits in taking a few simple precautions in purification, producing an antiserum and then testing it under the conditions in use and modifying it thereafter if necessary. In the example given, the problem of preparing IgG Fc portions is thereby avoided, although it must be admitted that an antiserum raised against such pieces of the IgG molecule would have a much higher degree of specificity to begin with and require less absorption for most assays. In some laboratories the procedures required for separation of the Fc pieces might be available, and in these instances there would be benefit in producing such a highly purified sample.

Using a purified or semi-purified immunogen, the next step is to decide on the type of animal to be immunized. Again, this will depend on the facilities of the investigator, although in general it is preferable for most workers to use the largest animals available. This is particularly the case where the assays of antibody are being carried out for diagnostic purposes, because in these circumstances one can expect a heavy work load and therefore a large demand for antiserum for the assays. To produce large volumes of good antiserum from small animals is difficult. The decision to be taken on the type of animal to be used should not be made on the basis of the efficiency of the response of the animal so much as the volume of antiserum which can be obtained. Although there are differences in the response of different species of experimental animals some of which will be discussed below, the major consideration has to be the question of available volume.

To take an example, let us consider the use of anti-human IgG in assays for *Candida albicans* antibody, which is a routine diagnostic service in our laboratories. For this assay 100 mg of antiserum (anti-IgG) protein produce about 30 ml of working reagent. The reagent will be used in a volume of about 100 μl per assay tube and therefore it is likely that about 200 sera could be assayed with one preparation of radiolabelled anti-immunoglobulin. (The remaining 100 tubes would be accounted for by controls and standards.) In a busy laboratory 200 samples per week would be expected, particularly where the assay of *Candida albicans* antibody is being used to assess the immune response of patients, in addition to those patients where the organism is thought to be producing a pathogenic effect. Thus, 100 mg of antiserum protein could be used within 1 week, and this might represent a volume of 2 ml of antiserum, therefore producing an annual requirement of 100 ml of antiserum. If we assume that to obtain 100 ml of antiserum we require the collection of approximately 250 ml of whole blood, it is clear that the bleeding of animals such as mice (where volumes of about 2 ml are reasonable at each bleeding), or guinea-pigs (where the collection of 5 ml is reasonable) or rats (similarly 5 ml) is tedious. Further, there is no doubt that assays which can be operated for several years with the same stock antiserum are preferable. The difficulties of assay caused by the different characteristics of the antiserum can be eliminated by the use of the same antiserum over long periods.

For these reasons, the investigator is advised to choose a species of animal which is capable of producing large volumes of blood at each bleeding.

The discussion which follows is based on our experience with sheep and rabbits. For the reasons above, it will be clear that sheep are to be preferred for the production of antiserum, but we recognize that rabbits are more commonly available for the experimenter, and a description of immunization of these animals, which we have used extensively, will also be provided.

Immunization of sheep

Dosage of immunogen

It is commonly assumed that a larger amount of antigen administered to an animal will produce a greater response from the animal. Although there is some truth in this reasoning and some associated experimental proof, there are a number of important qualifications.

A dose of immunogen which is too low will lead to tolerance, as will a dose which is too high. We have not defined the area of low-zone tolerance in sheep but our data suggest that immunizing doses of 50 µg are as good as doses of up to 1 mg of antigen. Thus, in terms of yield of antibody (i.e. amount) and specificity, doses of antigen of 50, 100, 200 and 500 µg and 1 mg have been comparable in our hands. However, it is easier to prepare, say, 50 µg of partially purified antigen than 1 mg and we therefore tend to use the lowest of this dose range.

There is also a theoretical advantage in adopting the lowest possible dose. Suppose that after partial purification the antigen is contaminated to about 5% by an unwanted substance (also an antigen). If a dose of 1 mg is used, the animal will receive 50 µg of the contaminating antigen, and this we know is capable of immunizing against the unwanted substance. If, however, 50 µg of the preparation is used, only 2.5 µg of contaminant will be injected and this may be too small an amount to induce a response. In a limited series using human IgG as the antigen we have evidence that antibody to contaminating IgA is produced with 1-mg doses but not with 50-µg doses. Of course, it is always possible to remove such unwanted anti-IgA activity by absorption of the antiserum, but the example is mentioned to illustrate the principle that the lowest successful immunizing dose should be used.

It is worth noting that doses of immunogen much lower than this are sometimes used, especially in rabbits, by cutting the precipitin line out of an agar gel and using this line (containing only a few micrograms or less of antigen) as the immunizing dose. This technique, which is applicable when the antigen is difficult to isolate, is successful because the antigen is complexed with antibody and the complexes are more immunogenic than antigen alone. The use of immune complexes for immunization purposes will be dealt with more fully below.

Route of immunization

Having selected the dose of antigen to be used, the next question is to decide on the route of injection. In sheep the possibilities are:
1. Intravenous.
2. Intramuscular.
3. Subcutaneous.
4. ? Intraperitoneal.
Here it is necessary to decide what kind of antibody (of sheep origin) is likely to

be optimal in the radioimmunoassay. As indicated already, the real test is to try the antiserum in an assay, but a few predictions are reasonable. Firstly, one requires the maxmimum amount of antibody per unit volume and this means that preferential stimulation of IgG is desirable. Secondly, antibody is required which has a high affinity for its antigen, and again the IgG formed in the 'middle' of a response will be desirable. Thirdly, it may be necessary, particularly in microbiological work, to avoid natural agglutinins to common organisms. These are almost always IgM antibodies and to avoid them it is convenient to use the IgG fraction from the sheep antiserum. Clearly this entails making sure that the sheep's response to the immunogen is IgG.

Intravenous injection of an immunogen tends to favour IgM responses. Classically, the production of (IgM) agglutinating antisera to bacteria and virus is achieved by repeated intravenous injections of increasing dosage. The injections must be repeated frequently because, after the first injection, the IgM already formed complexes with the antigen introduced and will neutralize it, unless there is a large antigen excess. Hence it is necessary to increase the dose at each injection to stimulate a further response. Although IgG is produced in such a response most of the antibody is IgM. This kind of regime is therefore not suitable for preparing RIA antisera, unless there is a specific reason for wanting to use an IgM antibody, which is unusual.

Both intramuscular and subcutaneous injections favour IgG production, probably because absorption of the antigen is delayed and the response therefore has time to change from IgM to IgG production. Intramuscular injection of sheep is, in our experience, the most suitable, and a convenient site is the gluteal muscle of the hindquarter. Only one injection site is necessary. A problem with subcutaneous injections is the formation of a granuloma at the site, which may ulcerate and become secondarily infected from outside. Granuloma formation also occurs with intramuscular injection—indeed it is probably a necessary component of a good response—but because the site is deep and enclosed, ulceration and infection do not develop.

As indicated above, the delay of the absorption of antigen increases IgG responsiveness, and this is one of the reasons for using an adjuvant with the initial injection of immunogen.

Adjuvants

Two adjuvants, Freund's complete and incomplete adjuvants, are commonly but not exclusively used in the preparation of antisera. Both of these prolong antigen absorption by inducing granuloma formation but probably have additional effects on the immune response. The granuloma formation is greater with Freund's complete adjuvant, which probably accounts for the fact that the response when using this adjuvant is considerably delayed beyond the 10–14 days which is seen with antigen alone. An optimal response with these adjuvants generally occurs after about 20–30 days. Both of these adjuvants are water-in-oil emulsions (see Appendix for details) formed by mixing the antigen-containing water phase with an oil (Dracheol) and Arlacel-A, which assists the emulsification. In addition, Freund's complete adjuvant contains killed *Mycobacterium tuberculosis*. The wax-D component of the cell wall of this organism has powerful adjuvant properties which are added to the effect of the water-in-oil emulsion.

Our standard procedure is to use Freund's complete adjuvant for the initial injection of antigen. Clearly, a considerable period is required to allow the primary response to be fully developed, and we routinely wait for at least 6 weeks when immunizing sheep before any booster injection is given.

Although the primary response is well established with these adjuvants, the amount of antibody produced is low and requires booster injections of antigen to produce the high levels of antibody necessary in the antiserum.

A booster injection can be given either in saline or in adjuvant (Freund's complete or incomplete) and, depending on the choice, by a variety of routes. For example, in saline the injection can be intravenous, intramuscular or subcutaneous, and with adjuvant either intramuscular or subcutaneous. It is not a good practice to administer these adjuvants intravenously.

Our own preference is for an injection of antigen in saline, intramuscularly, of the same amount as used initially to prime the animal. All that remains is to decide when to bleed the animal for the antiserum. We have found that any period less than 7 days or over 12 days after the booster dose is unsatisfactory. The secondary response, although vigorous, is short and sharp, and outside these limits inferior amounts of antibody will be obtained in the antiserum. If for any reason bleeding cannot be performed within 12 days, it is better to give another booster dose, wait for the desired period and then bleed.

Bleeding

Bleeding of sheep is best carried out by canulation of the jugular vein, using an 18 Intracath connected to a 'reversed' intravenous infusion set with the float chamber removed. The blood is collected into small-volume (20–25 ml) containers. The advantage of collecting 20 × 20-ml volumes instead of a single 400-ml volume is that a greater yield of serum is obtained using the smaller volumes.

It does not distress a sheep (adult, normal size) to lose between 400 and 500 ml at one bleeding, and the effect of this loss is to boost the antibody response further, so that another bleed 3 days later is often satisfactory.

If a longer period elapses before further bleeding it is better to boost the response of the animal, wait for 1 week, and then bleed. The animal can then be allowed to 'rest' for as long as a year, whereupon another booster injection and bleeding will produce a good antiserum once again.

It is often argued that to keep an animal for a year without using it is uneconomical, but this is not necessarily the case, especially if the antiserum produced is of high quality for RIA work. In the example given earlier we indicated that an RIA for *Candida* antibody might require 100 ml of antiserum per year. To buy this amount of antiserum would cost at current prices about £500–700, whereas the cost of maintaining a sheep for a year is generally less than £400.

Our practice has been to obtain several litres of antiserum over the initial period and then to keep the animal 'quiescent' for a year. If more antiserum is required, the animal is boosted and bled, but if there is no demand for antiserum the animal is boosted and bled out and the remaining serum stored. We have, rarely, boosted and bled an animal annually for up to 5 years, with excellent results as judged by the quality and consistency of the resulting reagent.

Immunization of rabbits

Dosage of immunogen

As will be noted from the above discussion, the doses of immunogens used for sheep are fairly low, considering the size of the animal to be immunized. Indeed, the doses are so low that to reduce them any further carries a risk that low zone tolerance may be induced. Accordingly, it is our practice to use the same range of immunizing doses for rabbits (50–1000 μg).

Route of administration

The initial injection should be given in Freund's complete adjuvant, intramuscularly into both gluteal regions. A refractory period of 4–5 weeks should be allowed before giving a booster injection.

It is sometimes argued that intramuscular injection even with Freund's complete adjuvant gives a poor response. Certainly, in our experience the response of rabbits to the same dose of immunogen (50 μg) presented in the same way (intramuscularly in adjuvant) in sheep and rabbits gives an excellent response in the former species and a poor response in the latter, although this may be due to differences in the performance of individual animals.

The critics of the intramuscular injection routes for rabbits often argue that the dose, suitably subdivided, should be given into the footpads of the hind feet of the animal. This is not easy to do without distressing the animal, and as granuloma formation proceeds the feet become seriously ulcerated and infected and a cause of discomfort to the animal. It is not our practice, therefore, to inject into the footpads and we feel that should this route be employed, the experimenter must watch for problems very carefully and treat the animals properly to minimize pain and suffering. Further, we know of no evidence which proves that immunization by this route (footpads) produces a better antiserum than intramuscular injection in adjuvant. The booster injection for rabbits should be given by intravenous injection, with the immunogen in saline (about a 1-ml volume is ideal) into the marginal ear vein. However, there is a risk of anaphylaxis occurring, although this is rare. To avoid this problem a small dose of immunogen (say 50 μg in saline) should be given intramuscularly to 'desensitize' the animal, followed by the intravenous booster dose a day later (again about 50 μg in saline). After 5 days the animal should be bled.

Bleeding

This is best carried out by section of the marginal ear vein. It is important to realise that the animal may have to be bled many times to make up the volume of antiserum required for RIA. Thus, apart from any consideration one may give to the welfare of the animal, it is in the interests of the experimenter to be as careful as possible in venesection, so as to preserve the vein for as long as is required. Several simple measures can be taken. Firstly, if bleeding is being carried out only to test the antiserum (and therefore a small sample is all that is required), it is advisable to take the blood with a small volume syringe (2–5 ml) fitted with a 25# needle. A dab of xylol (xylene) should be applied to the dorsal surface of the ear tip (point X in Fig. 3.1) to cause minor irritation and 'bring up the veins'. It is best to have two operators. One restrains the rabbit with the help of a suitable box, whilst at the same time holding the ear in a flat, forward horizontal position (see Fig. 3.1) gripping the ear at points A and B. This has the effect of closing both veins and thus engoring them. The vein should be entered as close to A as possible. If scarring results, the vein is entered at point

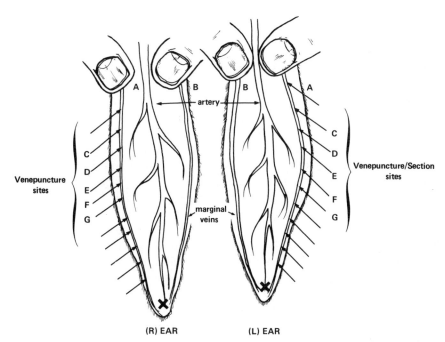

Figure 3.1. Diagram to illustrate the venesection sites of the rabbit ear (see text for details)

C on the next occasion, and so on. In this way it is possible for many bleedings to be taken before the vein is too scarred for further work. Thereafter, the same approach is applied to the other ear. It should be noted that simple venepuncture should not seriously damage the vein.

When a larger blood sample is required (the maximum at one session for the average rabbit is 30–50 ml), the same procedure is followed but the vein is cut neatly across with a sharp scalpel blade and the blood is allowed to drip into a container below. A thin layer of vaseline over the area to be incised assists the blood to flow.

When bleeding by either of these methods is complete the blood flow can be stopped by removing the pressure over points A and B and applying direct pressure through a ball of cotton-wool, at the entry or incision site. The xylol applied to the tip of the ear must be thoroughly removed by liberal washing with ethanol (or methylated spirit). If this precaution is not observed, drying, ulceration and infection of the ear will result.

Absorption of antiserum

Having obtained the antiserum, some absorption is usually necessary. However, if antiserum has been produced to highly purified fragments of an immunoglobulin this may not be the case. Otherwise, two forms of absorption will be needed.

To remove light-chain activity

Because the light chains are common to different immunoglobulin classes, any antiserum raised against any whole immunoglobulin molecule will cross-react with light chain antigens of other classes of immunoglobulin. This activity can be removed by absorption with purified light chains. The common source of light chains for such a purpose is urine from patients with multiple myeloma who have Bence-Jones proteinuria. There are two types of light chain, kappa (κ) and lambda (λ) and each individual myeloma patient will have only one of these type in the urine. It is usually necessary, therefore, to collect urine from several patients and test the light chain type. This can be done conveniently by immunoelectrophoresis on a concentrated sample of urine, using anti-κ and anti-λ antisera to develop the precipitin lines. It is possible, of course, to raise these antisera, although the amounts required for typing make it relatively uneconomical and it is probably preferable to purchase the required antiserum from one of the firms who supply it (see Appendix).

Having obtained preparations of light chains, the absorption can be carried out either (a) in the fluid phase or (b) using a solid phase. In the former method the antiserum is mixed in varying proportions with the light chain preparations for 2 h at 37 °C and 4 h at 4 °C. Any precipitate which forms is removed by centrifugation and the antisera tested to see whether cross-reactivity remains. This testing can be carried out by immunoelectrophoresis using the absorbed antiserum against the following: normal serum, purified IgG, IgM and IgA (all at high and low concentrations), and some of the light chain preparations which were used for absorption. Myeloma sera are a good source for preparing IgG, IgM and IgA for this purpose. The result should indicate that the antiserum is specific only for its intended immunoglobulin and has no demonstrable light chain reactivity which reacts with other immunoglobulins.

It should be noted that the absorption must not remove too much of the specific activity required. If it does, the antiserum is either deficient and should be replaced by an improved product or the light chains are contaminated by whole immunoglobulin molecules which have removed essential material. This is not uncommon because patients with Bence-Jones proteinuria often have a degree of renal damage which allows whole immunoglobulin molecules to pass into the urine (especially IgG). Thus, anti-IgG activity may be absorbed out of the antiserum. A careful check of the full protein content of a light chain preparation is therefore advisable before it is used for absorption. Alternatively, the light chains can be separated by chromatography on Sephadex G-200 or the method of absorption outlined below can be used.

It should be noted that even if absorption is followed by a satisfactory result in immunoelectrophoresis, the possibility of cross-reaction cannot be completely excluded, because the method is relatively insensitive. For most purposes, much of the cross-reactivity can be assumed to have been removed, and the antisera will usually perform well in routine diagnostic assays. For exacting work, however, it is recommended that a solid-phase binding radioimmunoassay be used to detect minor cross-reaction followed by further absorption if necessary. A solid-phase assay can be carried out using the absorbed antiserum radiolabelled with iodine-125 (see below) and tested against IgG, IgM and IgA (and if possible IgD and IgE) adsorbed to a solid phase such as cyanogen bromide-activated Sepharose® (see Chapter 2). Binding of the antiserum should be high with the specific Ig (e.g. IgG) and low with others.

Solid-phase absorptions can be effected by glutaraldehyde insolubilization of the protein or by linkage of the protein to a solid-phase matrix such as Sepharose®. The latter method is described in Chapter 2.

The glutaraldehyde treatment is as follows. The protein content of the solution to be treated is adjusted to between 300 and 400 mg/l and dialysed against 0.15 M NaCl (100 × volume) for 24 h. The dialysis is essential to remove free amino acids which would otherwise interfere with the insolubilization. The solution is buffered at a ratio of 1:10 with 1 M phosphate buffer at p.H 7.2 (see Appendix for buffer recipes) and glutaraldehyde [2.5% (v/v) in distilled water] is added at a ratio of 3:10. Insolubilization should occur quickly (within 10–15 min) but should be allowed to continue for about 1 h. The insoluble protein is then washed thoroughly in several changes of 0.15 M NaCl, by repeated dispersal of the insoluble material effected by drawing and expelling the material into a 20-ml syringe fitted with 25# needle. After washing, all surplus fluid is withdrawn and the antiserum added, mixed (by drawing through a syringe) and maintained for 2 h at 37 °C and a further 4 h at 4 °C. The mixture is then centrifuged and the absorbed antiserum removed and tested as described above.

The insoluble protein can be 'regenerated' for further use as an absorbent, by washing the protein with glycine–HCl buffer (pH. 2.4) (see Appendix) several times at 4 °C followed by several washes with 0.5 M NaCl at room temperature. The advantage of solid-phase absorption is that it does not lead to dilution of the antiserum, and this may be particularly important if the antiserum is weak and one cannot afford to lose any of the activity by dilution.

An alternative method of absorption independent of light chain preparations can be used if serum, depleted of the appropriate immunoglobulins, is insolubilized. Thus, in the case of anti-IgG antiserum, whole serum devoid of IgG can be used. To prepare sera without the major immunoglobulin components, the following methods are suggested.

Removal of IgG   This can be done conveniently by chromatographic separation using a QAE-A50 (Pharmacia Fine Chemicals) column. The starting sample of serum (5 ml) is equilibrated by dialysis overnight against a 'high' pH buffer (3.2 ml of diaminoethane + 4.25 ml of glacial acetic acid per litre of distilled water; pH 7.2) and run with the same buffer on a column of QAE-A50 (60 × 3.0 cm). The eluted sample, which contains the IgG, is collected and when readings of protein in the eluate are zero the buffer is changed to a 'low' pH buffer (6.1 g of anhydrous sodium acetate + 15 ml of glacial acetic acid per litre of distilled water; pH 4.0). The remaining proteins are eluted from the column, collected and concentrated by dialysis against Carbowax (mol. wt. 20,000), prior to dialysis and treatment with glutaraldehyde. It is important to check the material eluted at low pH for IgG by immunoelectrophoresis, prior to insolubilization and absorption.

The advantage of using this method is that antiserum activity against some non-immunoglobulin serum proteins will be removed in addition to light chain activity which is absorbed by the content of IgA and IgM contained in the eluate. The method is also useful for preparing IgG for immunization to produce anti-IgG.

Removal of IgA   This can be conveniently achieved by differential precipitation of IgA using zinc sulphate. Zinc sulphate (1 M solution) is added to a final concentration of 0.05 M to the protein solution (previously adjusted to a concentration of 30 g/l by spectrophotometry or some alternative method). After adequate mixing (2 h at room temperature) the material is centrifuged and the supernatant discarded. IgA-free serum is found in the precipitate, which is redissolved in 1% EDTA and dialysed, concentrated and tested by immunoelectrophoresis for the absence of IgA. If the product is satisfactory it is treated with glutaraldehyde and used as an absorbent (for anti-IgA antisera). The supernatant from the precipitation can be subjected to preparative electrophoresis to produce a preparation of IgA for immunization.

Removal of IgM   This is best achieved by chromatography on a Sephadex® G-200 (or equivalent) column. A suitable size of column is 80 × 2.5 cm and the sample is run on the column, eluting with 0.2 M phosphate buffer (pH 7.4) or Tris–HCl buffer (pH 7.3) (see Appendix). The 'early' protein peak contains most of the IgM, although it should be noted that some of the latter separates along with other immunoglobulins. To remove all of the IgM, repeated chromatography may be required. The samples eluting after the primary protein peak are collected, concentrated and then treated with glutaraldehyde prior to use as an immunoabsorbent (to purify anti-IgM antisera).

All of the above methods demonstrate the basic approach to absorption procedures for any antiserum. There are, of course, many other ways in which the same end can be achieved, but those given illustrate the principles involved.

To remove other cross-reacting antibodies

The sections above describe how to remove unwanted antibody activity which is directed towards immunoglobulins. However, the antiserum to be used in RIA may have activity against components which are not part of the normal serum, but which may interfere in the assay. Thus, if one wished to measure human antibody to antigen X it is important to make sure that the antiglobulin used (sheep or rabbit) does not have natural activity against antigen X. In many instances such a problem will not arise, but in the case of assays of bacterial antibody this is often a problem. The reason for the difficulty is that sheep and rabbits have bacteria in their bodies, or are exposed naturally to bacteria which may provide the target antigens in assays of human antibody. *Brucella abortus* is a typical example, as is *C. albicans*. Such unwanted natural antibody can sometimes be ignored because it will be delivered in the same amount to each assay tube, thus raising the background radioactivity without interfering with the basic differentiation of antibody in the human serum samples (see Chapter 5). It should be noted, however, that under these circumstances it may lead to a reduction of the sensitivity of the assay.

It is often preferable to absorb the antiserum against such microorganisms prior to use in the RIA. In general, absorption against bacteria is best carried out using equal volumes of packed bacterial cells and antiserum, mixing well at 37 °C for 2 h and then at 4 °C for 12–18 h before removing the antiserum after centrifugation of the bacteria. In most instances it will not be difficult to obtain the large amount of bacteria needed for such an absorption because culture of the organisms is generally straightforward. In the case of viruses, however, it may be extremely difficult to obtain a large amount of antigen (e.g. cultured cells containing the virus) for absorption purposes. In these instances resort to purification of the anti-immunoglobulin by affinity chromatography may be advisable.

Affinity chromatography

In the methods outlined above the emphasis was on removal of unwanted or cross-reactive antibody, leaving the specific (or desired) antibody in the antiserum in high concentration. In affinity chromatography one reverses this principle by separating the component required, anti-IgG for example, and washing away the remaining unwanted protein and immunoglobulin.

In the example below, the preparation of specific sheep anti-human IgG is considered. The first step is to prepare pure human IgG. This can be done by QAE-A50 chromatography (see above) or by DEAE-cellulose chromatography (Fahey and Terry, 1978). The pure IgG is linked to cyanogen bromide-activated Sepharose (see Chapter 2) and the Sepharose® is poured into a short column which is capable of being reversed. Sheep anti-human IgG is run through the column. The amount which can be handled on each column must be determined by trial and error, watching the outflow for the appearance of excess anti-IgG activity (detected by gel diffusion or immunoelectrophoresis). Once equilibrated, the IgG on the column will have attached anti-IgG. The column is washed with several volumes of a mild buffer (PBS, pH 7.2) until no protein issues from the column. This can be checked by spectrophotometry at 280 n.m. Elution of the antibody (anti-IgG) can then be achieved by reversing the column and applying either a low pH buffer (glycine–HCl, pH 2.4) or a high molarity salt solution (3.0 M potassium thiocyanate). The retrieval from such columns, in our experience, is better using the high molarity salt solution, although even with this only about 20% of the contained antibody is likely to elute. The reason for the low recovery is that antibody which has been specifically prepared to have high avidity is too strongly bound to the Sepharose® to allow removal without denaturation. Nevertheless, it must be recognized that even a small amount of antibody is extremely useful because it is *pure*. Accordingly, even though the amount is small, it will perform many assays and needs only a fraction of the radioisotope required if an 'impure' antiglobulin is used. The sensitivity of RIA using such purified antibody is usually high (*N.B.* the RAST system for assay of IgE antibody). The preparation of specific antibody in this way is strongly recommended, although it is appreciated that more work is needed to establish the assay. Where retrieval of antibody from the column is reasonable, it is of course possible to re-use the column (after washing) for the preparation of more antibody.

Recently, we have used two different eluents for affinity chromatography columns. The first, 50% ethylene glycol, removes approximately 60% of the attached antibody. The volume required to do this is usually the equivalent of two bed volumes of the column. The eluted material should be dialysed against several changes of a suitable buffer such as 0.1 M PBS (pH 7.2) for at least 24 h. Thereafter the antibody will be suitable for radiolabelling.

The other reagent is 0.5 M propionic acid. This elutes very efficiently, removing between 90 and 100% of the attached antibody. A dialysis step as above is also required. However, much of the antibody is denatured and the remaining activity after this type of separation is too low to be of value. It must be added, though, that the procedure is ideal for 'regenerating' a column prior to use again as an immunosorbent.

Use of staphylococcal protein A

Increasingly, many radioimmunoassays of antibody are being developed using staphylococcal protein A, instead of anti-immunoglobulin. This substance, a component of the cell wall of the Cowan strain of *Staph. aureus*, has the ability to bind human IgG (except for IgG$_3$). It can be obtained commercially in the purified form (Sigma Ltd.), or it can be refined in the laboratory (Mallinson et al., 1976). When radiolabelled, for example, using the Bolton and Hunter reagent (see below), the protein A functions in the same way as an anti-IgG and can be used to quantitate antibody of this immunoglobulin type. It must be remembered, however, that antibody of the IgG$_3$ subclass will not be detected by this reagent and, although this may not be a serious problem in most studies, it would clearly be so if antibody of that subclass was of interest.

Monoclonal antibodies

Introduction

Regardless of how well anti-immunoglobulin reagents are raised in animals, they have properties which are undesirable in a highly sensitive assay system for antibody. Such antisera are heterospecific and display heterogeneity of titre, affinity and classes of immunoglobulin. They usually require absorption and are available in limited supply, thereby adding to the problems of standardization and repeatability.

Monoclonal myeloma proteins have none of the problems of conventional immunoglobulins in that a large amount of chemically identical immunoglobulin molecules are produced. However, in nearly all cases, the antibody specificity of the myeloma protein is unknown. They are therefore excellent for immunochemical studies on the molecules, but of no use as diagnostic reagents. A series of elegant experiments by Kohler and Milstein (1975) has shown, however, that it is possible to fuse spleen cells from pre-immunized mice with cells of a mouse myeloma line to produce a 'hybridoma' line which secretes immunoglobulins characteristic of the myeloma proteins but with antibody specificity to the immunizing antigen. It is therefore theoretically possible to obtain self-perpetuating lines of cells which can easily be cultured *in vitro* and which secrete monoclonal antibodies of a predetermined and selected specificity.

The general technology involved in the production of monoclonal antibody is reviewed below.

Myeloma cell lines

Most hybridization studies have used a cell line P3-X63-Ag8, derived from BALB/c mice, which secretes IgG$_1$ and kappa chain. For antibody production, it is useful to use myeloma lines which have no inherent secretion of immunoglobulin to avoid production of non-antibody immunoglobulin (or peptides) which might interfere with the performance of the required antibody. For this reason P3-NSI-1Ag4-1, which is a myeloma line producing only kappa chain or X63-Ag8.653, a non-secreting line (both from BALB/c mice), are more useful. The above cell lines are 8-azaquanine resistant and will not grow in HAT selective medium.

'Immunized' spleen cells

Commonly, spleen cells from BALB/c mice immunized with the appropriate antigen are used. However, other strains of mice or even other species may be used successfully as spleen cell donors. Immunization schedules to induce antibody production in spleen cell donors vary considerably and the best method will presumably vary with each antigen. In the original experiments of Kohler and Milstein, the monoclonal antibody was of the IgM class but IgG antibody has been produced by using spleen cells from hyperimmunized mice. Thus, depending on the use of the hybridoma product, the immunization schedule may play an important role. If the antibody is to be used in a complement fixation test, IgM may be the preferred class because of its efficiency in complement fixation. On the other hand, if the antibody is to be used in a primary binding assay, IgG antibody may be more useful because of its molecular size, precipitation characteristics and the ease with which the Fc portion may be removed.

Hybridization

Kohler and Milstein fused the plasmacytoma cell and normal spleen cells using inactivated Sendai virus; subsequently polyethylene glycol (PEG) has been found to be useful for fusion. While the ideal parameters for fusion have not been firmly established it is usual to use PEG (mol. wt. 1000 to 4000 daltons), which is non-cytotoxic at a concentration of approximately 30% for 5–10 min. The myeloma cells and normal ('immunized') spleen cells are mixed for fusion in ratios varying from 1:1 to 1:10 and then dispensed into micro-titre plate wells (10^5–10^6 cells per well) in HAT selective medium. Cells which are not fused do not survive in this medium.

Cloning

After a suitable incubation period, the micro-titre plate wells containing viable cells should be screened for the specificity of their secretions. This procedure usually involves a primary binding assay (RIA or ELISA) and polyacrylamide electrophoresis, electrofocusing, peptide mapping or sequencing. Cells from wells containing antibody of the desired specificity should then be cloned. This is usually done by plating a limiting dilution of the cells on to a layer of 'feeder cells'. Following a suitable incubation period, the culture supernatants are checked for specificity as above using the primary binding assay. After establishing the appropriate clone it can be cultured 'en masse' in tissue culture, yielding 5–10 μg/ml of antibody or alternatively in live mice, producing 10–20 mg/ml of antibody in ascitic fluid.

Properties and uses

Monoclonal antibody is a homogeneous chemical reagent of very restricted specificity available in unlimited supply. This type of reagent is therefore valuable for standardization of immunological tests and is also a unique serological reagent for use in new tests and in the study of the pathology of disease. Monoclonal antibody will have very wide application in diagnosis and many research projects, particularly those involving the identification of antigens, hormones, cellular receptors, etc.

RAIOLABELLING TECHNIQUES

Iodination

The most convenient and widely used marker for protein in radioimmunoassay is radioactive iodine. Two commercially available isotopes, ^{125}I and ^{131}I, both emit gamma radiation, although ^{131}I is in addition a β-emitter. Gamma radiation can be measured directly through the walls of most assay tubes, whilst β-emitters such as ^{14}C or ^{3}H require the addition of a liquid scintillator and the use of special counting vials. Thus gamma radiation is more convenient, and as the chemical substitution of proteins with iodine is a relatively simple procedure, we routinely use ^{125}I in the radioimmunoassay of antibody. There are two reasons for using ^{125}I in preference to ^{131}I: (i) ^{125}I has a half-life of 60 days compared with 8 days for ^{131}I, and therefore the radioactive conjugate has a longer shelf-life; (ii) in addition to β-radiation, ^{131}I emits gamma radiation at a higher energy level than ^{125}I, and is therefore less desirable on safety grounds.

However, ^{131}I remains a useful alternative to ^{125}I, and indeed it is possible to use the two isotopes simultaneously in certain circumstances. Most gamma counters can discriminate between these isotopes by virtue of their different energy levels of radiation, and thus two different radiolabelled proteins can be measured independently in the same sample.

It is sensible to use no more radioactivity than is absolutely necessary for adequate performance of each assay, and all radioactivity should be kept in a defined area where contamination can be regularly monitored. In particular, the radioiodination procedure presents the greatest potential exposure to radiation, and this should be performed wherever possible in a localized area used for no other purpose, where any spills or leakages can be easily contained. An appropriate isotope labelling area together with some of the equipment required is shown in the photograph in Fig. 3.2.

Apart from safety considerations, low levels of radioisotope substitution minimize physico-chemical or radiation damage to the protein, and thus help

48

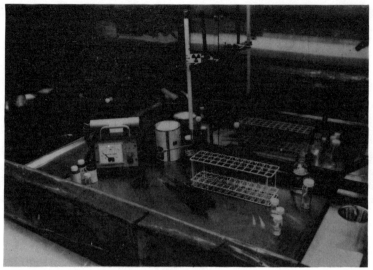

Figure 3.2. A radiolabelling area (see text and Appendix for details)

preserve its antigenicity or antibody activity. In the various antibody assays described in this book, each antigen–antibody system may require different levels of radioactivity substitution of the anti-immunoglobulin. At the lowest level of antibody to be measured in any particular assay, the sample radioactivity should be high enough to allow a reasonably short counting time. The degree of purification of the anti-immunoglobulin is also an important factor in determining the necessary level of radioactive substitution. In a crude globulin extract of hyperimmune serum, perhaps only 5–10% of the total immunoglobulin is antibody of the desired specificy. In these circumstances, 90% of the radioactive ^{125}I may be linked to immunoglobulin which is irrelevant to the assay, and is removed in the washing procedure. Purification of the antiserum prior to labelling, for example by affinity chromatography, will increase the proportion of radioactive iodine linked to immunoglobulin of the desired specificity, and so the total radioactivity required to produce the same final count rate will be less. (See earlier for antiserum purification procedures.)

Radioactive decay is a random process, and repeated measurement of the same sample will produce a Poisson distribution of results around the 'true' value. The standard error of a single measurement of n counts is $\sqrt{n}$, and so it can be calculated that for an acceptable error of (say) 1%, 10 000 counts must be collected:

$$\text{Error} = \frac{\sqrt{n}}{n} = \frac{100}{10\,000} = 1\%$$

In our laboratory, a sample count of 10 000 would be expected within 3 min or less. If the counting time is too long, e.g. 10 min or more, the advantage of rapid processing by radioimmunoassay may be lost. The specific activity of the anti-immunoglobulin must therefore be high enough to produce an acceptable count rate in the lowest activity sample. For practical purposes, the initial activity should be around three times this minimum value, in order to give the radiolabelled anti-immunoglobulin a shelf-life of 2–3 months.

Methods of radioiodination

The technique in commonest use for the radioiodination of proteins is that initially described by Greenwood et al. (1963), and later modified by McConahey and Dixon (1966). We have found this method to be rapid and reproducible and to have little deleterious effect on the antibody activity of the immunoglobulin which is being radiolabelled. The method employs chloramine-T as a oxidizing agent, producing $^{125}I^+$ in the reaction mixture, which then exerts an electrophilic attack on tyrosine residues in the protein. The reaction is stopped by the addition of a reducing agent (sodium metabisulphite), and finally potassium iodide is added as a carrier for excess of unreacted radioactive iodine. Protein-bound ^{125}I is separated from any remaining ^{125}I by gel filtration through a small column of Sephadex G-25. The reaction conditions represent a compromise between maximizing the efficiency of radiolabelling and minimizing damage to the protein. The labelling efficiency is related to the concentration of protein, the concentration of chloramine-T and the duration of the reaction (McConahey and Dixon, 1966; Greenwood et al., 1963). However, since chloramine-T is an oxidizing agent it can alter protein structure by reacting with amino acid chains, e.g. SH groups. Efficiency may therefore be sacrificed in favour of milder reaction conditions which are less damaging. Chloramine-T, as indicated above, oxidizes certain amino acids preferentially, these being tyrosine, tryptophan and phenylalanine. In fact, most of the effect is on tyrosine. The extent of labelling of a compound therefore depends largely on the amount of tyrosine contained. Clearly, the greater the number of tyrosine residues contained in the molecule, the greater will be the changes in that molecule and these may produce significant alterations of the biological activity of the substance. In the case of small molecules which are radiolabelled for use in conventional radioimmunoassays of 'antigen', e.g. hormones such as ACTH, this may be a serious problem because the high intensity may either change the reactivity of the antigen for its antibody or may cause a degree of 'primary radiation decomposition' (where structural damage to surrounding residues occurs as the isotope decays) which renders the material inappropriate in the assay.

Considerations such as these are not so important when one is labelling antiglobulin, which in radioimmunoassay of antibody is the usual product. Thus, most of the products to be labelled will be antibodies to immunoglobulins, raised in sheep, rabbits or some other species, and will in general be IgG or equivalent antibodies. IgG of mammalian origin contains 20–30 tyrosine residues per molecule but only 2–4 of these residues occur in the variable (i.e. antigen binding) region of the molecule. Indeed, there is a suggestion that the

50

tyrosine residues do not play a major part in the antigen receptor site. It is therefore possible to label the molecule heavily with iodine without serious interference with its antibody function (i.e. antiglobulin activity). With the method outlined above, levels of 1.0–5.0 μCi/mg of protein would be expected and it is unlikely that such a degree of labelling would seriously interfere with the antiglobulin activity.

Radiolabelling procedure with chloramine-T

The basic radiolabelling procedure used in our laboratory is as follows: 500 μCi of carrier-free [125]I (The Radiochemical Centre, Amersham, England) is dispensed in a small volume (10 μl) and 100 mg of protein (globulin fraction) in 2 ml of 0.1 M phosphate buffer (pH 7.4) is added. A 100-μl volume of chloramine-T (1 mg/ml) is added and the solution is mixed and left at room temperature for 5 min. The reaction is stopped by adding 100 μl of sodium metabisulphite (1 mg/ml) followed immediately by 100 μl of potassium iodide (5 mg/ml).

The above procedure provides a working guide which may be modified as circumstances demand (see original papers for details). The amount of ^{125}I handled at any one time should be kept to a minimum, and it may be possible to use less than 500 μCi if the antiserum is purified. If a purified anti-immunoglobulin has been prepared, smaller amounts of protein e.g. 1 mg, may be employed, in which case the amounts of chloramine-T and sodium metabisulphite are reduced in proportion.

When the reaction is complete, the radioactive mixture is applied to a Sephadex G-25 (coarse) gel filtration column (30 × 2.5 cm) and eluted with 0.1 M phosphate buffer (pH 7.4). There is little point in using expensive commercial columns for this purpose, as a crude separation is adequate and radioactive contamination may in any case limit the life of the column. Accordingly, we use 25-ml pipettes which have been sawn off at the top just below the neck, and fitted at the bottom with a small cotton-wool plug and an end-piece of 2–3 inches of rubber or plastic tubing. Such a column is packed with 5 g (dry weight) of Sephadex G-25 (coarse) pre-swollen for 30–60 min in phosphate buffer. Non-specific binding of labelled protein to the Sephadex may be minimized by first running 2 ml of bovine serum albumin [4% (w/v)] into the column and then washing it through with 50 ml of buffer. The radioactive sample can then be applied to the top of the column by pipette, and run into the gel. The column is eluted with buffer and 25-drop fractions are collected. To avoid contaminating valuable fraction-collecting equipment, we collect the fractions manually, moving tubes held in a stainless-steel rack beneath the column outflow. To prevent drops of radioactive material falling on the rack, it is useful to clamp the column outflow with a pair of Spencer-Wells forceps before moving from one tube to the next.

The radioactivity of each fraction can be determined either with a hand-held Geiger monitor or by withdrawing samples (10 μl) for each and measuring the radioactivity in a gamma counter. For the column and sample sizes described, a clear separation of protein-bound and free ^{125}I should be obtained within the first twelve fractions collected, as shown in Fig. 3.3. The fractions comprising the first (bound) radioactivity peak are pooled and diluted to 15–30 ml in 0.1 M phosphate buffer (pH 7.4). Labelled antiserum prepared in this way may be kept in Bijoux bottles which are stored in lead containers at 4 °C. Two or three drops of a 5% solution of sodium azide or merthiolate should be added to each Bijou bottle. A useful life of 6–8 weeks for these preparations is normal, provided that the initial specific activity is high.

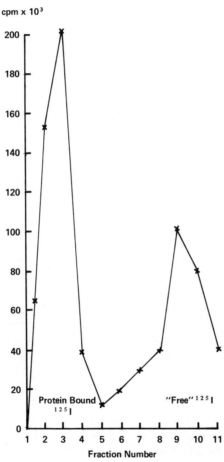

Figure 3.3. Separation of free and protein bound ^{125}I by chromatography with Sephadex G-25 (coarse grain). The column (35 × 1 cm) was eluted with PBS and fractions of 1 ml were collected. The counts are for 10-μl aliquots drawn from each fraction. The labelled protein was anti-human IgG

Other methods of radioiodination have been described and four of these are mentioned here, although we would only consider them after the chloramine-T procedure had been shown to be unsuccessful.

Lactoperoxidase method

In this method, the enzyme lactoperoxidase catalyses the iodination of tyrosyl residues, also requiring hydrogen peroxide as a substrate (Morrison et al., 1971). Contamination of the final radiolabelled product with lactoperoxidase can be avoided by coupling the enzyme to a solid phase such as cyanogen bromide-activated Sepharose (see Chapter 2) and removing this at the end of the reaction by centrifugation (David, 1972). There is some evidence that the lactoperoxidase method causes less denaturation than chloramine-T (Miyachi and Chrambach, 1972), and it may be worth trying in circumstances where the protein to be labelled is found to be particularly susceptible to oxidation damage.

Iodine monochloride method

This is an older method (McFarlane 1968; Ceska et al., 1971) which is a more complex and less efficient process than chloramine-T radioiodination. However, the method may again be less damaging to some proteins, and may be used if problems of denaturation are encountered with other methods.

Bolton and Hunter reagent

This method is useful if the protein does not contain tyrosine, or is seriously damaged by direct iodination (Bolton and Hunger, 1973). In the first stage, the chloramine-T procedure is used to produce ^{125}I-labelled 3-(4-hydroxphenyl)propionic acid N-hydroxysuccinimide ester. This reagent is an acetylating agent, and readily reacts with free amino groups on the protein. Thus it is possible to obtain a radiolabelled protein in which critical tyrosine residues remain intact.

Chloraglycoline method of Fraker and Speck (1978)

This is a modern and simple method which may replace the chloramine-T procedure in many laboratories. The active substance is 1,3,4,6-tetrachloro-3a,6a-diphenylglycoluril, which is insoluble in water, but can be 'plated' on to the surface of the reaction vessel from a methylene chloride solution, the methylene chloride being evaporated at 37 °C. The protein, radioactive iodine and potassium iodide are then added in borate–saline buffer (pH 8.2) and the reaction is allowed to proceed for 5 min at 0–2 °C. The reaction is stopped simply by decanting the mixture from the reaction vessel, thus avoiding the potentially harmful reduction step which terminates the chloramine-T method.

The results presented by Fraker and Speck (1978) suggest that under the mild reaction conditions employed, this method preserves antibody activity more effectively than the chloramine-T method.

Storage of iodinated materials

Aggregation

Aggregation of anti-immunoglobulin may occur during the radioiodination procedure and during storage. Repeated freezing and thawing is especially liable to aggregate globulin, and this should be avoided. Centrifugation of older preparations before use may help to remove insoluble aggregates, and soluble aggregates can be separated from 7S globulin by gel filtration through Sephadex G-150.

Radiation damage

Radiation damage is unavoidable, but can be minimized by reducing the degree of radioactive substitution to the lowest level consistent with the convenience counting of assay tube radioactivity.

Storage conditions

Our practice is to store radiolabelled anti-immunoglobulins as dilute solutions at 4°C, with sodium azide or merthiolate as bacteriostatic agents (to a final concentration of 0.05%). The solutions can be conveniently contained in Bijoux bottles, which in turn are placed in small lead containers:

Quality control of material

The two main requirements of the radiolabelled anti-immunoglobulin are that it should retain its antibody activity and that it should produce measurable levels of radioactivity at the lower limits of antibody detection. Thus, each batch should be tested against a reference serum in the assay, to ensure that a linear calibration graph (see Chapter 5) is obtained with a low level of background radioactivity. There is probably little to be gained from using sophisticated techniques to monitor the structural integrity of the labelled molecules, as in the context of the radioimmunoassay procedure the retention of biological activity is really all that is required. However, the following may be worthy of consideration.

Trichloroacetic acid precipitation

The integrity of the protein–isotope bond can be rapidly checked by precipitating the radiolabelled anti-immunoglobulin from solution by adding an equal volume of 20% trichloroacetic acid, and then measuring the percentage of radioactivity which is precipitated. Some degree of decomposition of the protein–isotope bond occurs during storage, and can be monitored in this way. If the washing procedures employed in the assay are adequate, it is unlikely that the free ^{125}I will lead to inaccuracies, but this will contribute to the reduction in specific activity of the anti-immunoglobulin.

REFERENCES

Bolton, A. E. and Hunter, W. M. (1973). The labelling of proteins to high specific radioactivities by conjugation to a ^{125}I-containing acylating agent. *Biochem. J.* **133**, 529–539.

Ceska, M., Sjodin, A. V., and Grossmuller, F. (1971). Some quantitative aspects of the labelling of proteins with ^{125}I by the iodine monochloride method. *Biochem. J.*, **121**, 139–143.

David, G. S. (1972). Solid state lacto-peroxidase: a highly stable enzyme for simple gentle iodination of protein. *Biochem. Biophys. Res. Commun.*, **48**, 464–471.

Fraker, P. J., and Speck, J. C., Jr. (1978). Proteins and cell membrane iodinations with a sparingly soluble chloramide 1,3,4,6-tetrachloro-3a,6a-diphenylglycoluril. *Biochem. Biophys. Res. Commun.*, **80**, 849–857.

Greenwood, F. C., Hunter, W. M., and Glover, J. S. (1963). The preparation of ^{131}I labelled human growth hormone of high specific radioactivity. *Biochem. J.*, **89**, 114–123.

Kohler, G., and Milstein, C. (1975). Continuous cultures of fused cells secreting antibody of predefined specificity. *Nature (Lond.)*, **256**, 495–497.

Kohler, G., and Milstein, C. (1976). Derivation of specific antibody-producing tissue culture and tumor lines by cell fusion. *Eur. J. Immunol.*, **6**, 511–519.

McConahey, P. J., and Dixon, F. J. (1966). A method of trace iodination of proteins for immunologic studies. *Int. Arch. Allergy*, **29**, 185–189.

Fahey, J. L. and Terry, E. W. (1975). Ion exchange chromatography and gel filtration. In *Handbook of Experimental Immunology*, Vol. 1, (D. M. Weir, ed.), Blackwell, Oxford, pp. 8.1–8.10.

McFarlane, A. S. (1958). Efficient trace-labelling of proteins with iodine. *Nature (Lond.)*, **182**, 53.

Mallinson, H., Roberts, C., and Bruce-White, G. B. (1976). Staphylococcal protein A; its preparation and an application to rubella serology. *J. Clin. Pathol.*, **29**, 999–1002.

Melchers, F., Potter, M., and Warner, N. L. (1978). Lymphocyte hybridomas. *Curr. Top. Microbiol. Immunol.*, **81**, 9–23.

Miyachi, Y., and Chrambach, A. (1972). Structural integrity of gonadotrophins after enzymatic iodination. *Biochem. Biophys. Res. Commun.*, **46**, 1213–1221.

Morrison, M., Bayse, G. S., and Webster, R. G. (1971). Use of lacto-peroxidase catalyzed iodination in immunochemical studies. *Immunochemistry*, **8**, 289–297.

Pinder, M., Musoke, A. J., Morrison, W. I., and Roelants, G. E. (1980). The bovine lymphoid system. III. A monoclonal antibody specific for bovine cell surface and serum IgM. *Immunology*, **40**, 359–365.

Steensgard, J., Jacobsen, C., Lower, J., Hardie, D., Ling, N. R., and Jefferis, R. (1980). The development of difference turbidometric analysis for monoclonal antibodies to human IgG. *Molec. Immunol.*, **17**, 1315–1318.

Tron, F., Charron, D., Bach, J. F., and Telal, N. (1980). Establishment and characterisation of a murine hybridoma secreting monoclonal anti-DNA antibody. *J. Immunol.*, **125**, 2805–2809.

Chapter 4

Precipitation assays

GENERAL ASPECTS

Assays of antibody which do not employ a solid-phase antigen will be considered in this chapter. In these assays a soluble radiolabelled antigen is used, which is first incubated with the test serum and then separated into antibody-bound and antibody-free fractions. If the radiolabelled antigen is initially present in excess, the amount of radioactive antigen in the antibody-bound fraction will give a measure of serum antibody activity. Because the assay is performed under conditions of antigen excess and because the reagent concentrations are low, the antigen–antibody complexes formed remain in solution. It will be evident that separation of bound and free antigen is a critical part of the procedure, a feature in common with the competitive-type radioimmunoassay used for the assay of hormones, drugs, etc. Separation methods in competitive assays have been reviewed by Ratcliffe (1974), and many could probably be adapted to the measurement of antibody. However, in practice the commonest method used for antibody measurement is the Farr test (Farr, 1958, 1971), in which the antigen–antibody complex is precipitated by the addition of ammonium sulphate to a final concentration of 50% (w/v). Unbound antigen remains in the supernatant.

THE FARR TEST

Principle

This technique is most readily applicable to the measurement of antibody to albumin, and was originally described for antibody to bovine serum albumin (BSA) (Farr, 1958). A concentration of 50% (w/v) ammonium sulphate at 4 °C precipitates serum globulin but not albumin, and therefore the only albumin molecules to be precipitated will be those which are specifically bound by antibody (globulin). The greater the antibody activity of the serum, the more radiolabelled albumin will be precipitated. Control tubes are included to

55

monitor (a) the total precipitable radiolabelled antigen by addition of tri-chloroacetic acid (TCA) and (b) non-specific precipitation of antigen in the absence of test serum. The format of a basic assay is shown in Table 4.1.

The Farr test has been applied to other antigen–antibody systems, the important considerations being that under the precipitation conditions used the antigen should be soluble and the antigen–antibody complexes should be insoluble and stable.

Modifications of the test have been used for the measurement of antibody to carbohydrate antigens isolated from Meningococcus (Gruss *et al.*, 1978) and Streptococcus species (Aasted *et al.*, 1979). The method is also in routine use for the measurement of auto-antibody to DNA in connective tissue diseases, particularly in systemic lupus erythematosus (Wold *et al.*, 1968).

One of the practical problems presented by the Farr test is that in order to measure the precipitated radioactivity accurately, the precipitate has to be washed free of all contaminating unbound antigen, and the tube itself must be drained thoroughly. A useful way of avoiding this has been proposed by Gotschlich (1971). In this method, ^{125}I-labelled antigen is used together with radioactive ^{22}Na, the latter being added to the antigen–antibody mixture as a volume marker. After precipitation of the antigen–antibody complexes in the usual way, a variable amount of supernatant is withdrawn and the radioactivity of either this or the remaining tube content is measured. Most gamma counters can discriminate between ^{125}I counts and ^{22}Na counts, although there is likely to be some spillage of ^{22}Na counts into the ^{125}I channel. The calculation of the percentage of antigen bound in each tube is as follows.

Spillover correction

Assuming spillover occurs in one direction only, count a sample of ^{22}Na in the absence of ^{125}I. If this has C counts in the ^{125}I channel and N counts in the ^{22}Na channel, then for each experimental sample:

$$\text{Corrected }^{125}\text{I counts} = {}^{125}\text{I channel count} - \frac{C}{N}(^{22}\text{Na channel count})$$

Using corrected values where appropriate,

let B be bound antigen count;

let I and N be total ^{125}I and ^{22}Na counts added, respectively;

let i and n be the ^{125}I and ^{22}Na sample counts, respectively, for either the supernatant or the precipitate + some supernatant, whichever method is used.

Supernatant only counted:

i = free antigen count in volume of supernatant removed

$= n/N(I - B)$

$Ni = nI - nB$

Table 4.1 General plan for the Farr assay

Serum dilution (0.5 ml)	1:10	1:20	1:40	1:80	1:160	1:320	Normal serum control	Antigen precipitation control	Total antigen count
N/10 normal serum	—	—	—	—	—	—	0.5 ml	0.5 ml	—
^{125}I-BSA	0.5 ml	0.5 ml	0.5 ml	0.5 ml	0.5 ml	0.5 ml	0.5 ml	0.5 ml	0.5 ml

Mix thoroughly and incubate overnight at 4 °C

	1:10	1:20	1:40	1:80	1:160	1:320	Normal serum control	Antigen precipitation control	Total antigen count
Saturated ammonium sulphate	1 ml	1 ml	1 ml	1 ml	1 ml	1 ml	1 ml	—	—
20% TCA	—	—	—	—	—	—	—	1 ml	—

All reagents and tubes should be kept at 4°C and mixed thoroughly as the addition is made. Leave for 30 min at 4°C, then centrifuge for 30 min at 2000 g and 4°C. Decant supernatants

	1:10	1:20	1:40	1:80	1:160	1:320	Normal serum control	Antigen precipitation control	Total antigen count
Re-suspend in 50% ammonium sulphate	3 ml	3 ml	3 ml	3 ml	3 ml	3 ml	3 ml	—	—

Centrifuge for 30 min at 2000 g and 4 °C and decant supernatant. The tubes should be left to drain and then the radioactivity of the precipitates measured in a γ-counter

$$B = \frac{Ni - nI}{n}$$

$$\text{Percentage bound} = \frac{100(Ni - nI)}{In}$$

Precipitate and some supernatant counted:

i = bound antigen + free antigen in remaining supernatant

$= B + n/N(I - B)$

$Ni = NB + nI - nB$

$$B = \frac{Ni - nI}{N - n}$$

$$\text{Percentage bound} = \frac{100(Ni - nI)}{I(N - n)}$$

This method avoids the need to wash the precipitate and drain the assay tube thoroughly, and has been usefully employed by Gruss *et al.* (1978) in a situation where variable amounts of supernatant were withdrawn from the assay mixture. However, in most instances it is probably more convenient not to use a second isotope but instead to measure accurately the volume of supernatant withdrawn and counted.

Calculation of results

The results are plotted as a graph of the percentage of antigen precipitated against the logarithm of the serum dilution. The antigen precipitation control (TCA tube) ensures that the radioactive label is attached to the antigen, and at least 97% of the added radioactivity should be precipitated in this tube (Farr, 1971). The normal serum control tube gives a measure of 'background' precipitation of free antigen, and can be subtracted from the sample precipitates (Osler, 1971). An alternative method of allowing for contamination of the precipitate with free antigen was described by Farr (1971), and is based on the assumption that the amount of contaminating free antigen in the precipitate is proportional to the free antigen concentration in the tube rather than to the total amount of antigen added. While this is probably true for 'non-specific' precipitation, normal serum is present in every tube as a diluent, and if it contains a low level of antibody itself, the effect would be constant in every tube including the normal serum control. The investigator must therefore decide which correction is appropriate for his own system.

Expression of results

The Farr test is conventionally described as measuring the antigen binding capacity (ABC) of serum at a given concentration. The serum dilution which binds 33% of the added antigen is determined, and all sera are compared at this precipitation point so that the antigen–antibody ratios will be comparable. As the weight of antigen which is precipitated at the 33% point is known, the weight which would be precipitated by 1 ml of undiluted serum can be calculated. This figure is the ABC-33, and a subscript is added to define the antigen concentration used. For example, if 0.03 μg of BSA is used as antigen, and 33% precipitation is obtained with 0.5 ml of a 1 in 160 dilution of antiserum, the calculation would be as follows:

$$\text{ABC-33}_{0.03} = \frac{\text{weight of protein}}{\text{precipitated}} \times \frac{\text{volume}}{\text{correction}} \times \frac{\text{dilution}}{\text{factor}}$$
$$= 0.01 \times 2 \times 160$$
$$= 3.2 \ \mu\text{g of BSA}$$

A distinction is made between the *antigen binding capacity* of the serum under the conditions of the assay and the *antibody content* in weight units. The antigen binding capacity is a function of both the antibody content of the serum and the avidity of the antibody for its antigen. A relative measure of the antibody avidity can be obtained by increasing the antigen concentration at which the assay is performed. If the antibody is of high avidity, a high proportion of it will bind antigen at the 33% precipitation level, even at relatively low antigen concentrations. An increase in the antigen concentration will produce little increase in the number of antibody molecules bound. In contrast, a low avidity antiserum would show a considerable increase in its ABC-33 as the antigen concentration is increased, as the law of mass action indicates that a higher proportion of antibody molecules would be bound to antigen. In his original paper, Farr (1958) demonstrated differences in the avidity of antisera obtained at various stages of the primary and secondary immune response by comparing their ABC-33 values with 0.02 and then 0.2 μg of BSA added as antigen.

A modification of the Farr test by Osler (1971) is said to measure antibody content rather than binding capacity. This method considers the limiting case when antigen is present in sufficient excess to bind all the antibody molecules, and the immune complexes precipitated will be of the form Ag_2Ab, assuming that only 7S globulin is involved. The weight of antibody binding a known weight of precipitated antigen can then be calculated as follows:

$$\text{moles of antibody} = \text{moles of antigen}/2$$

$$\frac{\text{wt. of antibody}}{\text{mol. wt. of antibody}} = \frac{\text{wt. of antigen}}{2 \times \text{mol. wt. of antigen}}$$

$$\text{wt. of antibody} = \frac{\text{wt. of antigen} \times \text{mol. wt. of antibody}}{2 \times \text{mol. wt. of antigen}}$$

The molecular weights of the antigen and antibody are best obtained experimentally by, for example, gel filtration methods, as published values may be misleading. Serum albumin in particular is liable to dimerize in solution and so may have a higher molecular weight than expected.

ADVANTAGES AND DISADVANTGES OF THE FARR TEST

The main practical disadvantage of the Farr test is that the precipitation procedure is inconvenient and time consuming, and limits the technique to those antigens which are soluble in 50% ammonium sulphate. In addition, as the radioactive label is attached to the antigen, any radioactivity which is present in the precipitate must be assumed to be antigen bound by antibody, and this might not be the case. In the measurement of anti-DNA antibody, for example, complexes of radiolabelled DNA linked to non-antibody protein, in particular Cl_q, can be precipitated under certain conditions of pH and ionic strength (Aarden et al., 1976). A further disadvantage of the Farr test is that it is not possible to measure antibody in different immunoglobulin classes, and so detailed information on the class specificity of the immune response cannot be obtained. In contrast, a solid-phase assay can differentiate between different immunoglobulin classes, and as it uses radiolabelled antiglobulin in the final stage of the test, only antibody molecules are detected. A solid-phase assay for anti-DNA has been developed using DNA adsorbed to plastic as antigen, and detects any (serum) antibody which binds to the DNA using a radiolabelled anti-globulin (Lange et al., 1976, 1978; Lange, 1978). This technique does not have the disadvantages of the Farr test outlined above, and has one further advantage. DNA cannot be readily substituted with iodine, and for use in the Farr test it is normally labelled with tritium, a β-emitter. In the solid-phase system, the antiglobulin reagent can be easily labelled with the gamma-emitter ^{125}I, and this has practical advantages (see discussion in Chapter 3).

Despite the disadvantages of the technique, new modifications of the Farr assay seem to work well. For example, using the modification of Gotschlich (1971), Gruse et al. (1978) have adapted the test to measure antibody to two different carbohydrate antigens of Meningococcus simultaneously. This test is done in microtitre plates with the antigens labelled with different isotopes of iodine, and the supernatant in each well is sampled for counting by dipping blotting paper into the wells. The Farr test is also well suited to the study of antibody avidity, as demonstrated in the original paper by Farr (1958). However, for most purposes we feel that a solid-phase assay offers practical and theoretical advantages in the routine measurement of antibody, particularly when, as is often the case, protein antigens are being used.

ALTERNATIVE PRECIPITATION METHODS

Other methods of precipitating the antigen–antibody complex have been employed, and may be useful where the ammonium sulphate technique is unsuitable. The second antibody method is commonly used in competition assays of antigen, and involves the use of an anti-human immunoglobulin prepared in some other animal species such as sheep, rabbit or goat. The anti-immunoglobulin cross-links the antigen–antibody complexes which are already in solution, and brings about precipitation. This method was one of the first used in antibody assay (Feinberg, 1954; Skom and Talmage, 1958) but has not been widely adopted since, although it has been applied to the measurement of anti-DNA antibody (Glass et al., 1973). It is important to calibrate this system so that complete precipitation is achieved throughout the range of (test) antibody levels being measured. Precipitation of antigen–antibody complexes is maximal when antigen and antibody are present in equivalent proportions and so it is necessary to ensure that anti-immunoglobulin is not added at too low or too high a concentration. This problem can be avoided by linking the second antibody to a solid phase, thus requiring only binding of the antigen–antibody complexes without their secondary precipitation. In this case, an excess of solid-phase anti-immunoglobulin is used.

In measuring anti-DNA antibody, Riley et al. (1979) compared the standard Farr technique with a similar method which used polyethylene glycol to precipitate the antigen–antibody complexes. These workers found that the latter method gave much higher values of antibody binding than the standard Farr technique, and they suggested that the polyethylene glycol method detects low avidity antibody which is dissociated from antigen during ammonium sulphate precipitation. An alternative explanation would be that polyethylene glycol is more likely to precipiate Cl_q bound DNA, and again the disadvantage of having the antigen labelled rather than the antibody becomes evident. Finally, as an alternative to any form of precipitation, Ginsberg and Keiser (1972) separated antibody-bound and free DNA by Millipore filtration, although it seems unlikely that this method could be easily applied to large numbers of samples.

REFERENCES

Aarden L. A., Lakmaker, F., and Feltkamp, T. E. W. (1976). Immunology of DNA: 1. The influence of reaction conditions on the Farr assay as used for the detection of anti-ds DNA. J. Immunol. Methods, 10, 27–37.
Aasted, B., Bernstein, D., Klopper, P. G., El Kholy, A., and Krause, R. M. (1979). Detection of antibodies in human sera to streptococcal groups A and C carbohydrates by a radioimmunoassay. Scand. J. Immunol., 9, 61–67.
Farr, R. S. (1958). A quantitative immunochemical measure of the primary interaction between I*BSA and antibody. J. Infect. Dis., 103, 239–262.
Farr, R. S. (1971). Ammonium sulfate precipitation of soluble antigen–antibody complexes. Methods in Immunology and Immunochemistry, Vol. 3, pp. 66–73. Edited by Williams, C. A. and Chase, M. W. Academic Press: New York and London.
Feinberg, R. (1954). Detection of non-precipitating antibody co-existing with precipitating antibody using I[131]-labelled antigen. Fed. Proc., 13, 493.
Ginsberg, B., and Keiser, H. (1972). A Millipore filter assay for antibodies to native DNA in sera of patients with systemic lupus erythematosus. Arthr. Rheum., 15, 438.
Glass, D. N., Caffin, J., Maini, R. N., and Scott, J. R. (1973). Measurement of DNA antibodies by double antibody precipitation. Ann. Rheum. Dis., 32, 342–345.
Gotschlich, E. C. (1971). A simplification of the radioactive antigen binding test by a double label technique. J. Immunol., 107, 910–911.
Gruss. A. D., Spier-Michl, I. B., and Gotschlich, E. C. (1978). A method for a radioimmunoassay using microtiter plates allowing simultaneous determination of antibodies to two non cross reactive antigens. Immunochemistry, 15, 777–780.

Lange, A. (1978). Evaluations of the simultaneous estimation of anti-ds DNA and anti-ss DNA antibodies for clinical purposes. *Clin. Exp. Immunol.*, **31**, 472–481.

Lange, A. Jacak, A., and Garncarek, D. (1978). Diagnostic specificity of autoantibodies: IV. A double antibody solid-phase radioimmunoassay for DNA antibodies—significance of ds DNA and ss DNA antibodies with test standardisation attempts. *Arch. Immunol. Ther. Exp.*, **26**, 893–897.

Lange, A., Roitt, I. M., and Doniach, D. (1976). A double antibody solid-phase assay for DNA autoantibodies for clinical use. *Clin. Exp. Immunol.*, **25**, 191–198.

Osler, A. G. (1971). Weight estimates of antibody based on antigen binding capacity. *Methods in Immunology and Immunochemistry*, Vol. 3, pp. 73–85. Edited by Williams, C. A. and Chase, M. W. Academic Press: New York and London.

Ratcliffe, J. G. (1974). Separation techniques in saturation analysis. *Br. Med. Bull.*, **30**, 32–37.

Riley, R. L., McGrath, H., Jr., and Taylor, R. P. (1979). Detection of low avidity anti-DNA antibodies in systemic lupus erythematosus. *Arthr. Rheum.*, **22**, 219–225.

Skom, J. H., and Talmage, D. W. (1958). Non-precipitating insulin antibodies. *J. Clin. Invest.*, **37**, 783–786.

Wold, R. T., Young, F. E., and Tam, E. M. (1968). Deoxyribonucleic acid antibody: a method to detect its primary interaction with deoxyribonucleic acid. *Science*, **161**, 806–807.

Chapter 5

Direct assays of antibody

INTRODUCTION

This chapter deals with the basic technology of the direct assay of antibody. In this method, the antigen is insoluble and may be either microorganisms (bacteria, viruses or fungi) or a soluble antigen which has been attached to a solid-phase adsorbent. The attachment of antigens to solid phases has been discussed in Chapter 2, and here it will be assumed that all the antigens are in an insoluble form.

The principle of the direct assay is illustrated in Fig. 1.8. Antigen is mixed with serum-containing antibody and incubated for about 30–60 min, usually at 37 °C. The mixture is thoroughly washed with an appropriate buffer and centrifuged and the supernatant is withdrawn and discarded. The washing procedure is repeated twice more and then radiolabelled antiglobulin is added to the pellet, mixed and incubated for a further 30–60 min. After this incubation the mixture is washed three times, the final supernatant discarded and the radioactivity of the pellet counted in a gamma counter. The incubation times and temperatures can be varied to a certain extent, although ultimately the antibody must be allowed to bind under reasonable conditions of time and temperature. The specificity of the antiglobulin used can also be varied (see below). If antibody is present in the sample under test, it will attach to the antigen and (unwanted) contaminating proteins will be washed away. The adsorbed antibody is then detected by attachment to it of radiolabelled antiglobulin. The greater the amount of antibody in the test sample, the more antiglobulin will be attached to the antigen, and the greater will be the subsequent attachment of radiolabelled antiglobulin. The amount of retained radioactivity will be directly proportional to the amount of antibody present in the sample. A control to which no serum is added provides an estimate of the 'background' binding of antiglobulin directly to the antigen or to the vessel wall.

If the assay is performed with several sera, each containing known amounts of antibody, or with dilutions of a single standard serum, a graph can be plotted of bound radioactivity against antibody content. Provided that antigen and antiglobulin are added in excess (see discussion below), the relationship between bound radioactivity and antibody content is linear. In practice, we prefer to plot the logarithm of the radioactivity against the logarithm of the dilution factor or antibody content, as shown in Fig. 5.1.

The advantages are:

1. Serial dilutions form a logarithmic progression in any case, and so the results of an assay of dilutions of a standard serum are readily plotted on semi-logarithmic graph paper.
2. Points become evenly spaced on such a graph instead of being clustered at the low antibody end. This prevents the highest antibody level point from receiving undue weighting in regression analysis.

Having constructed a linear standard graph, the antibody content of unknown samples can be obtained relative to that of the standard serum. The simplest approach to quantitation is to designate the standard serum as 100% or 100 units of antibody per millilitre, but the quantitation of antibody in weight units is preferable and will be discussed later. In a routine assay, results are better computed than read from a hand-drawn 'best fit' straight line through the standard points. Computation is done by linear regression analysis, and most

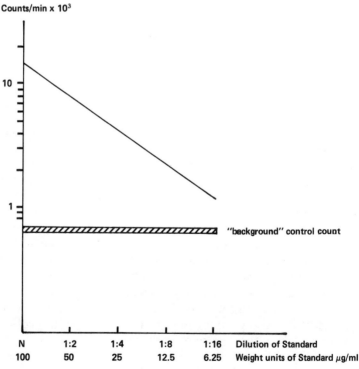

Figure 5.1. Regression line for assay of antibody, in a standard preparation, under conditions of excess of antigen and excess of antiglobulin

laboratories with access to even a small desk-top computer should have a suitable program as standard software. Statistical parameters such as the correlation coefficient or confidence limits for the estimate of an unknown sample can also be obtained with such programs, and these are often useful in assessing whether an assay is sufficiently precise for the purpose intended. A good account of the statistics involved can be found in the book by Snedecor and Cochran (1974) [see also Appendix].

The use of computing methods as described above can help considerably to process large numbers of samples. However, it is important to remember that a computer cannot improve upon the precision or accuracy of the data with which it is supplied.

It is our practice to plot manually the standard line for each assay before computation in order to maintain a subjective visual check on how well the assay is operating. This is particularly important for finding a 'plateau' (see below). The figures relating to such a plateau should not be fed into the computer unless a correction to exclude these has been added to the program. The technical factors which affect the assay are considered below.

AMOUNT OF ANTIGEN AND ANTIGLOBULIN

The relationship between bound radioactivity and the amount of antibody holds only if both antigen and antiglobulin are present in excess for each sample tested. If there is insufficient antigen some of the antibody will fail to become attached and will be lost in the washing process. The lost antibody will not be represented in the pellet at the end of the assay and the result will therefore be an underestimate of the true value. The same effect will occur for a different reason if insufficient antiglobulin is supplied. Although all of the antibody may be bound to antigen, a portion will remain undetected if there is not enough antiglobulin to bind every molecule of antibody. When an assay is established, it is therefore imperative that the conditions of antigen and antiglobulin excess are determined before any quantitation of samples is carried out. It will be clear that the conditions for samples with low levels of antibody will be less stringent than for samples with high levels. It is usual to test antigen/antiglobulin requirements with samples which have higher levels of antibody than any which can be reasonably expected in the routine performance of the assay. Although it is largely a matter of trial and error, the selection of a suitable standard antiserum which can provide an upper limit for the assay is essential (see below for detailed consideration).

Having selected a suitable standard antiserum, dilutions of the antiserum are assayed against a range of amounts of antigen, using a gross excess of antiglobulin in each tube. This procedure is expensive in reagents, but will be required only once for each assay system. Further, without this kind of titration, there is no proof that quantitation is possible. If antigen is not in excess the standard line as depicted in Fig. 5.1 will instead look like that in Fig. 5.2. At the highest concentrations of antibody there is a plateau which gives way to a linear

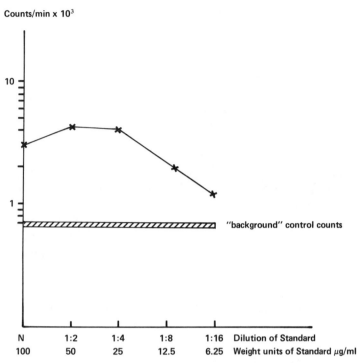

Figure 5.2. Regression line for assay of antibody in a standard preparation under conditions where antigen or antiglobulin or both are not in excess. Note that the 'plateau' at high antibody levels is not flat; it is typical that the neat serum has a lower value than the 1-in-2 dilution

decrease in radioactivity as lower concentrations of antibody are reached. Such a graph indicates that sufficient antigen exists for some of the antibody concentrations, but not for the highest. An antigen concentration is chosen which gives a straight line with no deviation from linearity at higher antibody levels. The procedure is then repeated using this antigen concentration with different amounts of radiolabelled antiglobulin to determine the amount which is in excess for the standard serum, but which is not too extravagant in terms of antiglobulin.

It should be noted that it is not possible to tell by simple inspection of a non-linear standard graph whether it is antigen or antiglobulin which is insufficient—indeed, it may be both. This can be deduced only in a trial and error fashion by altering the amounts of first one and then the other.

For two reasons a simple numerical excess of antigen and anti-globulin molecules over antibody is not enough to ensure a linear standard graph. Firstly, antigen should be present in gross excess to minimize the possibility of low avidity antibody remaining unbound, through lack of effective competition with more avid antibody. This ensures that the assay measures the amount of antibody rather than its biological activity. Secondly, the radiolabelled anti-globulin must attach to the bound antibody at a constant valency throughout the assay range for the standard line to remain rectilinear. There must therefore be enough antiglobulin not only to bind all the antibody molecules at high antibody levels, but to do so in the same antigen/antibody ratio as found at low antibody levels.

Unless such preliminary titrations are carried out, there can be no guarantee that antibody is being quantitated at all. This can be illustrated by reference to the plateau graph in Fig. 5.2. Antibody at a concentration 50 μg/ml records a count of 12 000/min, whereas it should give a count of 18 000/min according to the 'correct' standard line (Fig. 5.1), an underestimation of about 60%. At higher antibody levels the underestimation is even greater. Despite these seemingly obvious effects, most reports in the literature which use direct radioimmunoassays of antibody fail to indicate that the necessary preliminary titrations have been carried out, and for this reason the results are at best dubious, and at worst are not believable. It may be, of course, that the preliminary work is done but not reported, but in our opinion this work is so important that it must be mentioned in any investigation which uses the method. In the absence of adequate titration of antigen and antiglobulin requirements the method is no more accurate than the serological procedures which it replaces (e.g. complement fixation tests or agglutination test).

When the conditions of antigen and antiglobulin are correct, the resultant counts of radioactivity will be proportional to the amount of antibody contained in the serum (reference serum in this case). The range over which antibody can be measured will depend on the antibody level of the reference serum itself. Thus, when an assay is established it is necessary to decide the range which one requires. For most clinical usage, the range must be wide so that samples of differing values are successfully assayed in the same test. In Fig. 5.3, for example a typical farmer's lung radioimmunoassay for IgG antibody reveals that the assay range is from 6 to 400 μg/ml (see Chapter 7 for details of farmers' lung assays). The distribution of results usually found in farmers' lung is shown in Fig. 7.1 and it will be seen that few samples occur at the upper extreme of the range. However, these few samples will be inadequately tested and will require repeating after dilution to bring them within the assay spectrum. Samples at the lower end are almost always 'negative' in respect of disease and therefore to obtain an accurate answer is not important.

The situation may be different in research work. It may be necessary to have accurate quantitation of the lowest antibody levels, or of the highest, and in these circumstances the conditions of assay should be changed to achieve the required result. At the upper end of the assay range, the problems are solved by increasing the amount of antigen and antiglobulin to avoid any 'plateau' effect, or by diluting the sample and re-assaying under the same conditions. It must be recognized that sera with very high levels of antibody may still remain outside the range and this is particularly likely if the dilution chosen is small. Further, any dilution which is made may introduce error. Another option is to assay a

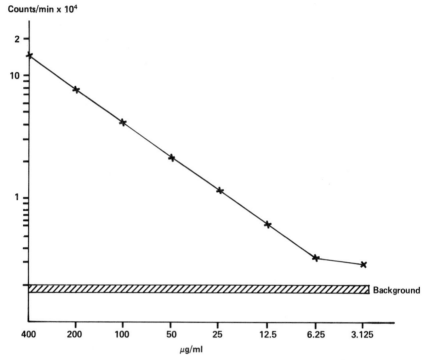

Figure 5.3. Typical regression line for assay of human IgG antibody to *M. faeni* (farmers' lung) showing the range over which the assay will work

smaller volume of serum. For example, if the initial estimation is made on 100 μl of serum, a reduction to 10 μl may bring the sample into the assay range, and one therefore has to assess whether it is easier (and more accurate) to dilute the sample or to pipette a smaller volume.

The problems of assay at the lower end of the range are different and are essentially due to the difficulty of distinguishing the low levels of activity from 'background' or non-specific attachment of the radiolabelled antiglobulin. It is essential, therefore, to consider the mechanisms by which such 'non-specific' attachment can occur, and the basis of the problem is shown in the results of an assay for IgG antibody to *Candida albicans* (Table 5.1).

The results from Table 5.1 are shown in graphical form in Fig. 5.4. The graph is linear with a good slope and there is no plateau effect, but the radioactivity obtained with an eight-fold dilution is not much greater than the background activity detected by the blank control tubes. Quantitation below the 1 in 8 level is therefore inaccurate because the radioactive count in these samples is high when compared with 'natural' background, that is, the count in the environment at the time of enumeration, and if the 'non-specific' binding could be reduced it should be possible to measure levels below the 1 in 8 dilution. Removal of most of the interfering activity is possible by using one or more of

Table 5.1   A set of results obtained with a RIA for human IgG
C. *albicans* antibody, using dilutions of a standard serum
illustrating the effect of absorption of the sheep anti-human
IgG with this organism

Serum concentration	Before absorption (counts/min)*	After absorption (counts/min)*
Neat	77 000	72 000
1 in 2 dilution	64 000	59 000
1 in 4	52 000	48 000
1 in 8	42 000	39 000
1 in 16	35 000	32 000
1 in 32	36 000	26 000
1 in 64	32 000	22 000
Blank control	34 000	18 000
Natural background	1 000	1 000

*Figures rounded to nearest thousand.

the methods indicated below. The term 'non-specific' is in some cases a mis-
nomer for the attachment may be either (a) specific but unwanted, or (b) true
non-specific activity.

REMOVAL OF SPECIFIC (BUT UNWANTED) BINDING

This activity can be explained in the example given (Table 5.1) by considering the origin of the anti-human IgG. In this case the antiserum was prepared

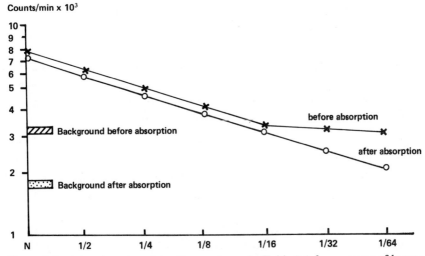

Figure 5.4. A log–log plot of the figures shown in Table 5.1 for an assay of human
IgG antibody to *Candida albicans*, to show the linearity

in a sheep, and it is therefore possible, indeed likely, that the animal had contact with *Candida albicans*, or with other fungi which share antigens with Candida species. If this is so, the animal will have antibody which reacts with the organism and this will be antibody of the type loosely referred to as 'natural'. Because a crude preparation of the sheep's antiserum (to IgG) was radiolabelled (a gamma-globulin preparation), the natural antibody would be included and would be radiolabelled with antibody of the 'desired' specificity. In the assay the unwanted sheep anti-Candida antibody attaches directly to the antigen (Candida cells) and produces a high background. The activity can be removed by absorbing the antiserum with Candida either before or after radiolabelling, and this can be conveniently done with packed Candida cells. (For further details of absorption procedures, see Chapter 3.)

It will be noted (Table 5.1) that even after absorption of the unwanted activity in this way, considerable attachment of antiglobulin remains in the control tubes. This is due to non-specific absorption of the antiglobulin by either the antigen or the test-tube within which it is contained, and its removal is considered below.

Before leaving this section it is worth noting that some of the binding to all samples (see Table 5.1 and Fig. 5.4) is removed by the absorption. The linearity of the line is maintained, however, dilutions of 1 in 16 and 1 in 32 now give meaningful results and it is possible that even a dilution of 1 in 64 may be accurately quantitated. Keeping in mind the fact that this assay is of a standard serum, with a concentration of 80 μg/ml, this change means that a range from 2.5 to 80 μg/ml is measurable, whereas the equivalent prior to absorption was 10–80 μg/ml. It is clear that 'background' interference is a major cause of failure to assay low levels of antibody satisfactorily.

REMOVAL OF NON-SPECIFIC ACTIVITY

The amino acid residues of proteins are 'sticky' by nature, owing to a large number of charged side chains, which interact electrostatically with antigens, and this causes them to attach non-specifically. It is important to note that some of the *sample* proteins which are antibodies of a different specificity from those reactive with the organism may attach in this way. The attachment may be reduced by one or more of the following procedures.

Increase in washings

Because the non-specific attachment is weaker than the specific attachment of antibody to its antigen, further washing should remove the former, leaving the latter intact. An increase from three to six washings usually reduces the background count, although there is a reduction also in the count of the reference samples because some of the specific activity, of low avidity, and some non-specific activity in these samples are also removed.

Addition of detergent

The inclusion of a detergent in the washing buffer reduces non-specific attachment of proteins. Commonly used materials are Tween 20 at a concentration of 0.5% (v/v) or Triton X-100 at 0.5% (v/v). The latter is the stronger and may remove considerable amounts of the specific activity also, and it is wise to see whether the weaker detergent will produce the desired reduction in non-specific attachment before proceeding to use Triton X-100.

Addition of a competing protein

The logic here is to add a protein to the wash buffer, which will saturate any sites available for the non-specific attachment of protein. The material used should (i) be easily available (ii) have a high degree of attachment and (iii) not interfere with the assay, i.e. have no cross-reactivity with either antigen or immunoglobulins. Suitable proteins are human or bovine serum albumin, both of which possess the above attributes. They are incorporated into the buffer at concentrations between 0.1 and 2%. It is axiomatic that the antiglobulin must be free of anti-albumin activity, but this is not difficult to arrange (see Chapter 3).

It is worth noting that the 'blank' control in some direct assays often gives a higher reading than the lowest standard serum dilitions, and this often disturbs the investigator. The phenomenon is due to the effect of serum proteins preventing, by competition, the non-specific attachment of the radiolabelled antiglobulin. Even with high dilutions of the standard serum there will be sufficient protein present to inhibit the non-specific attachment. In the 'blank' sample there is no protein in the first stage, so that antiglobulin in the second stage is bound to attach vigorously.

It is useful in most assays, therefore, to include a serum control which is known to have no antibody to the antigen being tested, for this will contain sufficient protein to inhibit the non-specific attachment of antiglobulins and will give a true 'blank' reading (see later for details of control for direct assays).

Variation of pH

Owing to changes in the charges on amino acid side chains, proteins attach differently to materials under different pH conditions. This is useful in the ELISA technique and in some radioimmunoassays where a solid-phase antigen is produced by attachment of the protein to plastic tubes or wells at pH 9–11. Conversely, proteins can be eluted from various materials by lowering the pH and, as described in Chapter 3, it is possible to remove antibodies specifically bound to their antigens by such a manoeuvre. Removal of non-specific binding in direct assays may be similarly possible by lowering the pH (from physiological), although the problem of removing specific activity must also be considered.

Variation of ionic strengths

As already described, non-specific attachment is usually due to electrostatic interaction between charged groups. This can be minimized by increasing the ionic strength of the wash buffer, e.g. by using phosphate buffer in 1 M Nacl.

By all of the above methods it is possible to produce assay conditions which are optimal for any assay of antibody which one may wish to measure. There are other technical aspects in the performance of these assays which are important, and which if ignored may lead to poor or erroneous results. These are described below.

TECHNICAL CONSIDERATIONS IN DIRECT ASSAYS

General

The performance of the assay must be precise if the results are to be good. If this seems naive, so be it; the fact is that attention to detail in the performance of RIA makes it possible to utilize its high sensitivity and reproducibility. In theory, an RIA should be 100% accurate. Given that the qualifications above with respect to antigen, antiglobulin excess and background limitation have been observed, the amount of attached radioactive tracer should reflect the amount of antibody present. This is subject to one qualification, that of valency change (see below), but this need not be a consideration here. It follows that any observed error is almost always due to technical error in the performance of the assay, and this can be considered under the following headings.

Pipetting and diluting errors

Samples, test or standard, have to be pipetted into containers for assay. If the pipetting error is 20%, which it may be with glass pipettes operating at small volumes, the reproducibility can never be less than 20% and is often higher because of other factors, such as those described below. Bearing in mind that RIA can and should operate with small amounts of sample (10–100 μl), and the fact that it is often used where reagents are difficult or expensive to obtain, the use of volumes outside this range is unusual. Therefore, 'standard' manual glass pipettes are not ideal. A better choice is the use of displaced-volume pipettes of fixed or variable volume such as the Eppendorf and Finn pipettes. These have disposable tips and can, in the hands of an experienced technician, be accurate to 5% or less at volumes down to 20 μl. An alternative is to use an electronically monitored automatic pipetting system which should be accurate to within 1% at volumes of 10 μl or less. These are, of course, expensive and may not be justified with a small workload. Such machines are available from several manufacturers (see Appendix). Whichever system is used it is important that the technician is 'stable' to the particular assay; by this we mean that he or she should have time (several months at least) to work with a particular assay. There is no doubt in our minds that if this is so, a technician will, after seeing the results of assay, continue to adjust and improve his or her performance whether this be manual, semi-automatic or fully automatic. (It is often forgotten that a fully automatic machine has to be loaded, primed and adjusted and that these are human functions which can, if incorrectly performed, lead to error.) We have frequently seen technicians, after months of RIA work, disconsolate at a result which for many would be more than satisfactory, and we cannot emphasize more strongly the point that most errors in RIA are human errors, and with careful selection of staff and adequate training they can be avoided.

As a consequence, any dilution required to produce either a standard curve or for re-assay of a high antibody sample (see above) must be made meticulously. There is no point in making dilutions with an error of 30% if the rest of the assay has an inherent error of 3%; but we have seen this happen. The method of making the dilutions can be varied, but we would recommend that it be either:

1. in large volumes (i.e. larger than needed for the assay) with accurate glass pipettes, or preferably
2. in small volumes with accurate displaced-volume dispensing pipettes. It is worth noting that the accuracy of these should be checked periodically by dispensing, say, twenty 50-μl volumes of water into a previously weighed container and making sure that the dispensed weight is close to 1 g (1 ml of water = 1 g at 4 °C).

Washing

From the discussion above, it is clear that adequate washing is essential if the problem of non-specific binding is not to interfere with the results of assay. However, it must also be remembered that any solid-phase material lost during the washing process will not be available for detection. If, for example, the assay is for detection of antibody to a bacterium, any bacterial cells which are lost during the first stage of washing (i.e. prior to the addition of antiglobulin) will be lost with antibody adsorbed to them, and therefore that antibody will not be subsequently available for detection. The same applies to the washings carried out after the addition of radiolabelled antiglobulin.

Before considering this aspect further, it is worth noting that assays using antigen bound to the surface of plastic tubes or wells are not apparently subject to this problem. The wash buffer can probably be completely evacuated from the container without fear of removal of the directly attached antigen and antibody. With bacterial suspensions, however, there are several important technical points, particularly with manual washing. If the assay is being carried out in tubes, the best method of washing is to resuspend the cells by using a vibrating mixer (e.g. Rotamix, Vibromix) and then to add a volume of buffer which is approximately half the total volume of the tube. In our laboratories we use 3-ml tubes, 1–1.5 ml of buffer being added after the preliminary mixing. This volume of buffer need not be accurately determined and can be dispensed from a pipette or a plastic disposable syringe. A multi-dispensing syringe (Cornwall syringe) is valuable for this. The contents of the tube are again mixed and the tube is filled with buffer and centrifuged. The speed and time of centrifugation must be pre-determined for each assay to produce a pellet of material which is complete and compact. If some particles remain in suspension they will be withdrawn, discarded and lost, leading to error. Some antigens, particularly those attached to large particles such as Sepharose® are easily deposited by light centrifugation for a short period, whereas others, e.g. Brucella microorganisms, require 2–3000 g for 10 min for adequate deposition. After centrifugation the supernatant is removed, usually by means of a Pasteur pipette coupled to a Venturi vacuum extractor attached to the mains water supply. All of the supernatant should be removed without disturbing the antigen pellet, and this requires experience. Thereafter the washing cycle is repeated at least twice.

A simple precaution to prevent removal of antigen during washing is to fit an adjustable stop to the withdrawing pipette so that it cannot be inserted so far into the tube as to make contact with the antigen. Another way of overcoming the problem is to use an automatic device which will dispense the buffer, mix the contents, centrifuge and then withdraw the supernatant. Instruments such as these are termed 'Coombs washers', and have two basic drawbacks: they are expensive, and they usually have a low capacity in terms of the number of tubes handled, often too low to make them of value for routine RIA work. Further, dismantling the apparatus to remove contaminating radioactivity is difficult. If the assay uses an antigen attached to the plastic surface of a well or plate, the washing is easier because loss of antigen usually does not occur. Automatic washers for such techniques are available, and are not too expensive. They dispense, mix and withdraw buffer in a single rapid cycle, usually dealing with ten tubes or wells at a time. (The names of the manufacturers of the washers are given in the Appendix.)

Storage of samples

Bacterial contamination of serum samples for RIA is a serious problem which may not be familiar to those used to more conventional immunological tests. The problem arises for two major reasions:
1. Microorganisms which are allowed to grow in a sample will be commonly occurring ones with which most humans and animals will have had continuous contact (notable amongst these are the staphylococci). It follows that the test samples and/or the antiglobulin are likely to have antibody to these organisms. When the samples are dispensed, the organisms growing within the serum are also dispensed, and during the test will be centrifuged with the true antigen particles (this does not apply to assays using plastic-bound antigen). Antibody will attach to the particles (it may be attached at the time of dispensing) and will, of course, act as a target for radiolabelled antiglobulin. The recorded radioactivity of the pellet may be due to such antibody–contaminant combinations, when no antibody is present in the sample against

the real antigen. Thus a false positive result is produced and in our experience this, together with the second problem below, are the only instances in which false positives occur in RIA of antibody.

2. A variation of the above is caused by the fact that contaminant microorganisms will degrade the proteins (including globulins), leading to aggregation. Aggregates of globulin will, of course, be deposited in the pellet and will bind radiolabelled antiglobulin, thereby producing a false positive result.

Contaminated sera can be 'cleaned' by ultracentrifugation or ultrafiltration prior to assay, but this is time consuming and it is better to process and store samples carefully to avoid contamination. In our view there are two main options. After rapid separation of sera (certainly within 6 h), they can be stored:

1. *Frozen*, either at −20 or −70 °C, until used for assay. There is one problem with freezing sera: if repeated assay of a sample is required (as it is for a standard serum), the freezing and thawing will lead to a reduction in antibody activity due to denaturation of the immunoglobulin molecules. In our experience, this effect becomes obvious after two or three freeze–thaw cycles and thereafter the antibody activity reduces by about 20% at each cycle. If it is necessary to repeat assays on the same sample, the sample should be frozen in the form of many small aliquots (say 0.2 ml), one of which can be removed at the time of each assay. In this way the bulk of the material is stably maintained at constant temperature.

2. *Refrigerated at 4 °C*. This popular method is very useful, but it must be remembered that some contaminating microorganisms can grow at this temperature, although slowly. With long-term storage, contamination can be serious. To avoid the difficulty it is wise to add a preservative such as 5% sodium azide to a final concentration of 0.05% to all stored samples.

Containers for assay

Antigen for direct assay of antibody is either (a) particulate or (b) soluble rendered insoluble by attachment to some type of solid phase (see Chapter 2). For the former category it is convenient to use test-tubes to contain the materials during assay. Glass test-tubes have the advantage of not adsorbing proteins non-specifically to the same degree as plastic tubes. However, they are more expensive are obviously breakable (a hazard with radioactivity) and require decontamination and recycling, which is also expensive. Plastic tubes are cheap, easily available and can be discarded at the end of the assay. A problem to be aware of is that approximately one in twenty (plastic) tubes has a flaw which can open on centrifugation, spilling the radioactive contents and causing contamination of the centrifuge. Such flawed tubes can be detected at the time of setting up the assay by careful examination. A further problem, utilized in some assays, is that proteins will absorb well to plastic and hence the non-specific activity increases. However, it is always possible to reduce this effect (see above). In our view plastic tubes are ideal for direct assay of antibody and we use tubes approximately 71×1.2 cm in size, which are easy to work with and which hold adequate volumes for washing.

For the second category of assay, i.e. insolubilized antigens, the choice of container is limited. Antigen attached to plastic requires either a plastic tube, or the well of a microtitre plate. A recent alternative is the use of plastic spheres 3–5 mm in diameter, which can be processed in tubes as for Sepharose®, and whose performance characteristics are good. Antigen attached to Sepharose® can be used either in a well or a tube, as can antigen attached to a cellulose paper disc (see Chapter 2).

STANDARD ANTISERUM

A standard antiserum should be selected which gives a linear regression line appropriate to the range of antibody levels anticipated. The choice of standard will vary with the particular assay. In clinical work it is advisable, after preliminary tests, to select a patient with a high level of antibody, and to obtain as much antiserum as possible from this patient. This serum must be carefully stored. A donation of one unit of clotted blood (releasing approximately 150 ml of serum) should standardize most assays for many years. If it is not possible to obtain a single large sample, an alternative method is to pool several smaller samples, all of which contain high levels of antibody.

Quantitation of antibody in standard sera

Many published radioimmunoassay methods measure antibody semi-quantitatively. For example, the commercial Phadebas RAST® kit (Pharmacia) classifies IgE antibody levels in grade 1–4, while other methods record the highest serum dilution which provides a radioactive count significantly above background (Friedman et al., 1979). We feel that the radioimmunoassay technique offers the opportunity for a more precise antibody quantitation than conventional serology, and if this is not fully exploited, much of the advantage of the method over other techniques is lost. Hence, we have stressed the need for a linear standard graph against which unknown samples can be assessed. Expressing the results as a percentage of the standard serum is a useful way of obtaining a relative measure of antibody levels in different sera, but the units of measurement remain arbitrary. For this reason we have attempted to standardize our assays to measure antibody in weight units. If this method is followed it allows different laboratories to compare results directly. Two different methods of standardization which we have employed are described below.

Agglutination assay

This is used to establish the amount of antibody contained in the standard serum. The assay requires large amounts of reagents to bring the antibody into a measurable range, but is usually only required once or twice during the working life of a standard.

Table 5.2. Diagram of the sequence of processing of a quantitative agglutination assay

A Antigen added to dilutions of standard serum (neat to 1 in 32) in 1-ml volumes → Washing →

B Cell pellets treated with glycine–HCl buffer → Supernatant measured for protein

C Antigen added to 1-ml volumes of saline (no serum added) → Washing →

D Cell pellets treated with glycine–HCl buffer → Supernatant measured for protein

E Antigen added to dilutions of standard serum (neat to 1 in 32) in 1-ml volumes → Washing →

F 1 ml of radiolabelled antiglobulin added to each tube → Radioactivity established for each tube → Washing → Cell pellets treated with glycine–HCl buffer → Supernatants removed and radioactivity determined → Radioactivity in cell pellets established

A series of tubes is set up according to the plan in Table 5.2. Four sets of tubes containing dilutions of standard from neat to 1 in 32 in approximately 1-ml volumes and a *gross* excess of antigen (1 ml of 5% suspension) are incubated for 1 h at 37 °C and 15 min at 4 °C, with frequent mixing. The amounts of reagents will vary in different systems but the volume of standard chosen should contain at least 0.5 mg/ml of total antibody (see below). Another set of duplicate tubes contains antigen only. The contents of the tubes are washed thoroughly but carefully. The pellets of cells from two of the rows (A and B) are then treated with Glycine–HCl buffer (pH 2.4) (1 ml per tube) whilst the tubes are held in an ice-bath. Rows C and D, containing only antigen, are also treated in this way. After 15 min the tubes are centrifuged at 4 °C and the supernatant is withdrawn, buffered with 0.5 ml of 0.2 M Na_3PO_4 and retained for the measurement of absorbance at 280 nm in a UV spectrophotometer. The values obtained for tubes in the C and D series (antigen only) are deemed to represent the amount of protein eluted by the buffer from the antigen, and this value is subtracted form the readings obtained for the rows A and B. The corrected values for the latter two rows of tubes represent the amount of antibody eluted from the cells at different dilutions of the standard serum, and when these values are plotted graphically against the dilution the resulting line should be rectilinear. If it is not, antigen excess has not been achieved and repeat assay is advisable. If, however, the plot is rectilinear it is possible to determine the amount of *total* antibody which has been eluted from the standard serum and therefore to deduce the amount it contained originally.

The quantitation of eluted antibody by spectrophotometry can be regarded only as an approximation, because the antibody will be heterogeneous and will include classes and subclasses all of which have different molar absorptivities. Our policy has been to use the molar absorptivity for human IgG (12.8) as the approximate value, on the grounds that most of the eluted material will be IgG and the influence of other Igs in changing this value will be small. Thus one can work from an absorbance reading in the supernatant to a weight of antibody (12.8 absorbance units = 10 mg/ml). Despite the obvious defects of this method, it is probably better than using a 'unitage' system as described above.

The limitation of the agglutination method is that the glycine–HCl buffer does not remove all of the absorbed antibody. However, using the remaining sets of tubes (rows E and F) the mixture of antibody and antigen is processed in the usual way for RIA and an excess of radiolabelled antiglobulin (about 1 ml per tube of the usual preparation) is added and allowed to incubate. After washing (normal RIA procedure), the radioactivity remaining in each pellet is measured in a gamma counter. This gives the total, bound radioactivity. The tubes are then eluted with glycine–HCl buffer in the same way as series A–D, and the radioactivity of the supernatant and of the pellet is measured. These two values should approximate to the value obtained for the pellet prior to elution. If they do not, error must be suspected and the test should be repeated. If there is agreement between the results, it is possible from the results for pellet and supernatant radioactivity to determine the percentage of antibody which remains attached to the pellet after the elution. (It has to be assumed that the antibody to be quantitated in the standard will behave in the same way as the antiglobulin during the elution.) A correction can then be applied to the values determined for rows A and B. Typically it will be found that the acid buffer elutes 70–80% of the adsorbed antibody, a much higher figure than that quoted in Chapter 3 for the preparation of specific antibody by affinity methods. The difference is probably due to the avidity of the various preparations. Correction of the figures for rows A and B according to this result gives a value for *total* antibody eluted. However, this is made up of IgG, IgM, IgA antibody, as well as (possibly) IgD and IgE, although in most work the last two can be ignored. Establishment of the relative concentrations of IgG, IgM and IgA in the eluted material can be difficult, and should be performed with sensitive RIAs set up for this specific purpose. However, it is recognized that such a facility is not usually available and the alternative that we have frequently used is to pool the concentrated eluates (from the neat samples) and to assay this pool using Mancini single radial immunodiffusion plates, specific for each of the three immunoglobulins. These assay plates have to have a high sensitivity and for this purpose we have been satisfied with 'low-level' Immunoplates.

An alternative to the use of Immunoplates is to apply the eluted material to chromatographic columns (see Chapter 3) and separate the IgM, IgG and IgA prior to quantitation by spectrophotometry using the correct molar absorptivities for each class of immunoglobulin.

Comparative method

A radically different method of quantitation which we have used recently attempts to carry out the whole procedure without separating the antibody from the antigen. It is best described by considering the quantitation of IgG antibody in a standard serum.

IgG is separated (see Chapter 3) and accurately quantified, by freeze-drying and weighing. A known weight of IgG is then reconstituted (e.g. about 1 mg) and radiolabelled with ^{131}I. It is important to monitor the fractions from the Sephadex G-25 separation column (see Chapter 3) for protein content (by spectrophotometry) and for radioactivity. This is because none of the IgG must be lost or, if it is, that amount must be known so that it can be deducted from the total amount of IgG which has been added to the column. After the separation it should be possible to know how much IgG is available, the volume in which it is contained and its radioactivity. Inevitably, this part of the method will involve contaminating the spectrophotometer cuvettes and other equipment, and these must be carefully decontaminated later. Further, there is more handling of isotope than in a straightforward RIA and care must be taken.

The radiolabelled IgG, is then bound to approximately 1 g of Sepharose® (see Chapter 2) using the normal procedure, and the percentage bound is determined by counting the radioactivity of the resulting product. (As a check it is useful to measure the radioactivity of the supernatants during the binding

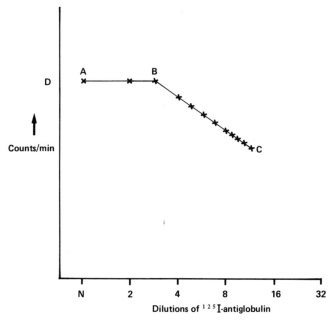

FIgure 5.5. Diagram showing the type of results obtained by titrating ^{125}I-anti-IgG against a constant volume of Sepharose–IgG (see text for details)

procedure, which will represent the unbound IgG.) From all of this information the amount of IgG bound to the Sepharose® can be established in weight units (e.g. μg IgG/ml of solid phase). This material is then used in the first of two assays.

Constant volumes of the Sepharose–IgG are mixed with dilutions of ^{125}I-labelled anti-IgG, and processed by the usual RIA method. The dilutions should be as narrow as possible, e.g. neat, 1 in 2, 1 in 3, 1 in 4, etc. The resulting radioactive counts (for ^{125}I) will define the conditions of attachment of the anti-IgG, as shown in Fig. 5.5. Between points A and B on this graph there is is no increased binding of anti-IgG as its concentration increases. Therefore, the antigen (Sepharose–IgG) is saturated. Between B and C, however, the linear regression indicates that the antigen is in excess, and that all of the anti-IgG added is being bound at each dilution. At point B the amount of anti-IgG added is 'equivalent' to the antigen concentration used. Suppose that the antigen has been used in 5-μg amounts. At point B the anti-IgG can fully bind 5 μg of IgG, and with a count of D cpm. Having established this, the second assay is run, using a dilution of antiglobulin appropriate to point B (i.e. 1 in 3 in this example), and dilutions of the standard serum (which is to be quantitated) mixed with an excess of the appropriate antigen. A typical set of results would be as shown in Fig. 5.6. In this representation, the dilution of standard 1 in 16, produces a count of D cpm. Hence this dilution will contain 5 μg of IgG.

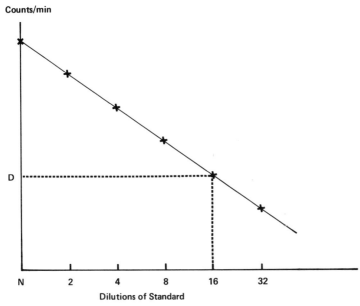

Figure 5.6. Diagram to illustrate the quantitation of antibody in a standard serum. Compare with Fig. 5.5 (see text for details)

Assume that 100 μl of each dilution have been used in the assay. The content of IgG antibody in the neat standard is therefore $10 \times 16 \times 5 = 800$ μg/ml.

There are several variations possible with this method of quantitation and we have presented the basic outline, in the hope that individual workers will adapt the method to their own purposes. Although the technique sounds cumbersome, it is probably technically easier than the agglutination method described above, particularly if several standards have to be quantitated. It must be realised, though, that the quantitation has to be rapid once the reagents have been prepared, because delays will reduce the radioactivity and lead to errors. The method is therefore best suited to analysis of several 'standard' sera at the same time, but has the additional advantage that antibody of other immunoglobulin classes such as IgD or IgE might be measurable, which would not be the case with the other method.

Other direct assays of antibody

Throughout this book the reader will find reference to variations of the basic direct assay technique described above. It would not be useful to consider all these variations in detail because they perform in much the same way as the basic method, and they are subject to the same limitations and errors. For example, it is just as important to take care with antigen and antiglobulin excess, correct washing techniques, buffers, etc. One variation is discussed briefly below to illustrate the kind of changes which are possible.

82

Double antiglobulin methods

Assays using two different antiglobulins can sometimes be more convenient than the basic direct RIA. Suppose that it is necessary to quantitate human IgM, IgG and IgA antibody to an antigen. Using the basic method three antiglobulins, anti-IgM, anti-IgG and anti-IgA (all prepared in rabbits, for example) have to be radiolabelled. This is expensive, and increases the hazard because more isotopically labelled antibody has to be stored. In a double anti-globulin assay, the rabbit anti-IgM, rabbit anti-IgG and rabbit anti-IgA would be used unlabelled and, after incubation and washing, radiolabelled sheep anti-rabbit gamma-globulin would be added.

The specificity of such a test is maintained because the sheep anti-rabbit will bind to the antigen only if rabbit antiserum has been bound, and the latter will bind only if human antibody of the appropriate immunoglobulin class is present. It is necessary, of course, to carry out the assays for different classes in separate sets.

A further advantage with this kind of approach is that it is not species-restrictive. In other words, the sheep anti-rabbit reagent can be used with rabbit anti-guinea pig IgG, rabbit anti-mouse IgG, etc. For veterinary work where antibody measurement is required in several species of animal, this is an important consideration. It is also worth noting that in many laboratories diagnostic work in humans goes on alongside research work in animals, and here again the use of a single, good, radiolabelled antiglobulin may be useful.

Apart from convenience, the double antiglobulin method has another advantage. This is an increased sensitivity which is due to an amplification of the number of radiolabelled molecules attached to the primary antigen–antibody complex. The discrimination of this kind of triple layer method is usually greater than that of the straightforward double-layer direct RIA.

However, there are disadvantages. In particular, the determination of anti-globulin excess is difficult because each antiglobulin must be separately and then conjointly titred with the antigen–standard system. Secondly, controls must be carefully devised to cover the possibility of either of the antiglobulins reacting with the antigen directly, and as a corollary to this (see earlier section) absorption of both antiglobulins may be necessary.

ADVANTAGES AND DISADVANTAGES OF RIA OF ANTIBODY

Advantages

There are a number of advantages of primary binding RIAs over conventional serological assays for the detection of antibody. Firstly, RIA is more sensitive than conventional methods and this is particularly true for the liquid-phase radioimmunoassays. Primary binding assays are more sensitive than serological tests which rely on secondary phenomena for the measurement of antibody, because antibody is not always capable of complement fixation, agglutination or precipitation (see Chapters 1 and 7). In addition, the assays which rely on a secondary reaction are subject to an error of at least 100% because doubling dilutions are required for titration of sera. The latter restriction inevitably means that a 2-week period between the first and second samples of serum is required for diagnosis, in order that antibody will increase sufficiently to pass these limitations. (Chapter 1). This period is shortened with primary binding assays, which detect movements, up or down, in antibody levels, after smaller time intervals (see Chapter 7 for a full discussion).

Secondly, primary binding assays are usually highly specific because of the ability to detect small changes in antibody level and because of the low error and the fact that they are not antagonized by anticomplementary components of serum, a haemolysed serum, or (in most instances) by the high lipid/lipoprotein contents of sera.

A third advantage of primary binding assays includes their ability to measure each class of antibody separately or, by dual labelling, in pairs. Rather than using a broad specificity antiglobulin reagent, antisera specific for the heavy chain of each immunoglobulin class may be used on duplicate samples. This is valuable in the study of the immune response to microorganisms and also provides a better picture of the status of an infected patient. If IgM antibody is found to be predominant the patient is probably in the early stages of infection, whereas high IgG or IgA levels usually indicate convalescence or recovery from the infection. Similarly, the separate measurement of antibody of different subclasses can provide information on the contribution of these to the immune response and perhaps indicate their involvement in recovery, or relapse and antigen clearance. Direct RIA is also well suited to the measurement of immunoglobulins in excretions and mucosal secretions and therefore provides an insight into local immune responses.

In addition to the versatility of direct RIAs there is also increased sensitivity because the final measurement depends on enhancing the number of antiglobulin molecules bound, which will be greater than the number of antibody molecules bound (see above). The sensitivity may be further amplified by the use of an antiglobulin reagent with a radiolabel to detect immune complexes. It is also useful to be able to select the class of antibody measured to the exclusion of non-specific binding (see Chapter 8).

A fourth attraction of solid-phase assays is the ability to select antigens by binding of highly specific antibody to the matrix, followed by interaction with a mixture of antigens. This allows retention of desirable antigens on the matrix with the exclusion of unwanted materials. This modification is advantageous in that parts of an antigen may be selected for study, provided that an antibody to the antigen has been prepared, and it removes the necessity for continuous purification of antigens by allowing crude preparations to be used. This type of assay, the remainder of which is conducted as a regular solid-phase assay, is particularly useful in the study of the immune response to viruses as specific antigens (e.g. group-specific, capsule or envelope), as these are often present in relatively small concentrations in a mixture of tissue culture cell antigens. The method clearly depends, however, on the development of a good antiserum which will bind the appropriate antigens.

A fifth advantage of primary binding assays is their accuracy. Various reports agree with the authors' experiments that a 12.5% between-tests variability and a 14% day-to-day variability are the maxima expected for RIA. The error would be similar for other primary binding assays, but considerably less than, for instance, the complement fixation test, which may vary up to 200% between tests. The reliability observed is achieved in spite of the rapidity with which a RIA may be performed. Provided that antigen is available, an RIA performed manually may be completed in approximately 4 h, including enumeration, and an operator may perform 1200–1500 tests per day (excluding enumeration). A manual complement fixation test, on the other hand, takes about 24 h with most antigens (including estimation of haemolysis) and an operator can handle about 120 samples per day, whereas an automated complement fixation test can process approximately 1000 samples per day. In other words, manual primary binding assays may be completed as quickly as automated complement fixation tests.

Finally, the radioisotopes commonly used for RIA are molecules of low molecular weight. Therefore, they can be used to label antigens of low molecular weight where other labels (e.g. enzymes) would be too large and would cause steric hindrance, or interfere with the specificity of reaction. Thus a radioactive label is of particular value with fragments of viruses and haptens, drugs, etc.

Disadvantages

There are a number of physical disadvantages to the use of any radioisotope. Thus, the most commonly used tracer for RIA is iodine-125, which has a half-life of about 60 days and which therefore cannot be stored for long periods. This can lead to standardization problems, which can be minimized in experimental work where sera may be collected and stored before assaying them all at the end of the experiment. The difficulty has, however, to be overcome in diagnostic work especially with assays which are continuous. On the other hand, enzyme-labelled antiglobulins (for ELISA) may be stored indefinitely in a frozen state with no measurable loss of activity. This disadvantage of trace iodination may be overcome by using an isotope of longer half-life such as tritium, carbon or radioactive sulphur, but these isotopes are not easily bound to antigens except *in vivo* and their 'soft' emissions can lead to loss of sensitivity of the RIA.

Further disadvantages of the RIA include the health hazard of manipulating the isotope and the continuous need for monitoring of the exposure of the operator. In the same context, though, this disadvantage of the RIA is diminished when contrasted with the dangers of substrates used in enzyme-linked antibody assay (ELISA), some of which are carcinogenic.

A problem alluded to elsewhere in the book is that RIA requires expensive enumeration equipment while other primary binding assay reactions may be estimated by visual inspection or by the use of less expensive equipment.

Finally, a disadvantage of all primary binding assays is interference due to autoantibody to immunoglobulins. This difficulty is most apparent when assay of IgM antibody is being attempted in sera which contain rheumatoid factor. In this instance IgG antibody may be attached to the antigen and will act as a target for the rheumatoid factor (an IgM autoantibody specific for human IgG). In the final stage of the assay any rheumatoid factor bound in this way will be detected by radiolabelled anti-IgM, even though the rheumatoid factor is not specific for the antigen used. It is, therefore, good practice when assaying IgM antibody to test for rheumatoid factor first, or to absorb the sera, briefly, with glutaraldehyde-insolubilized normal globulin.

GENERAL PLAN FOR DIRECT RIA OF ANTIBODY

This chapter finishes with a general plan of a representative assay, which should indicate the elementary design necessary. Modification, of course, will be necessary as work on any assay proceeds.

		^{125}I-antiglobulin
Neat standard serum	100 μl	+
1 in 2 standard serum	100 μl	+
1 in 4 standard serum	100 μl	+
1 in 8 standard serum	100 μl	+
1 in 16 standard serum	100 μl	+
1 in 32 standard serum	100 μl	+
1 in 64 standard serum	100 μl	+
Samples: X	100 μl	+
Y	100 μl	+
Z	100 μl	+
etc.		+
Blank control (no serum)	100 μl saline	+
Negative control (normal serum)	100 μl	+
'Standard' control	100 μl	

All samples receive 200–300 μl of antigen and are processed identically.

Normal sera for controls should be taken from healthy donors and should be shown to have no antibody in repeated assays. The 'standard' control is usually a dilution of the 'standard' serum not represented in the sequence, e.g. 1 in 10. Its antibody content is known, and if this value is not achieved against the particular run of standard dilutions it will be clear that the assay is not performing properly. Only when the 'standard' control accurately reproduces its known value can the assay be considered satisfactory.

REFERENCES

Friedman, M. G., Leventon-Kriss, S., and Sarov, I. (1979). Sensitive solid-phase radioimmunoassay for detection of human immunoglobulin G antibodies to varicella-zoster virus. *J. Clin. Microbiol.*, **9**(1), 1–10.

Snedecor, W. G., and Cochran, W. G. (1974). *Statistical Methods*. 6th ed. Iowa State University Press, Ames, Iowa.

Chapter 6

Measurement of total and specific IgE antibody by radioimmunoassay

GENERAL COMMENTS

IgE antibody is responsible for many cases of allergic disease in Western countries. This type of antibody (reaginic antibody) has a receptor which allows it to bind to mast cells. If the bound antibody then combines with the antigen which stimulated its production, activation of the mast cells occurs, and release of histamine and other vasoactive amines follows. It is the latter which produce the symptoms of disease and these are manifest as asthma, eczema, rashes or in extreme cases anaphylaxis. Allergic reactions producing these conditions are common, variously estimated as occurring in 5–15% of the population. Thus it is not surprising that methods for investigating the immunological basis of allergic disease have been pursued vigorously. Further, there are deficiencies in the traditional methods of investigation, i.e. skin testing and provocation testing. Consequently, attempts have been made in the last 10 years or so to measure the level of IgE antibody to incriminated antigens and to relate this to the clinical state of the patient, with a view to diagnosis and more efficient management of the condition. This chapter discusses the methods available for the measurement of IgE and their relative merits. In this discussion the term 'allergen' is used synonomously with 'antigen' and indicates only that an allergic response has occurred to such an antigen.

INTRODUCTION

The estimation of reaginic antibodies in the clinical laboratory is at present dominated by the availability of commercial kits to estimate IgE levels. The time involved and the technical expertise needed to carry out the measurement of total and specific IgE antibody levels using the kits is minimal, making it possible for most laboratories with access to a gamma counter to offer the service. The range of available commercial allergens for IgE antibody testing is comprehensive but is not as great as those for skin testing. IgE antibody kit estimations are available from Pharmacia Diagnostics Ltd. (see Appendix), and are of two kinds, one which measures the total IgE level in serum (Phadebas IgE PRIST®) and the other which measures IgE antibody to specific allergens (Phadebas RAST®). RIST (radioimmunosorbent test) is another method for total IgE measurement (see Fig. 6.1.).

It should be remembered that the PRIST and RAST tests are direct radioimmunoassays and can be successfully operated using items which may be prepared in the laboratory, if the staff expertise is available and the facilities are adequate. Further, it is of use to remember that the commercial kits can serve as a basis for modifications and improvements to meet one's own requirements, which may include the preparation of different allergens from those which are commercially available.

The main problem in any assay of IgE antibody is that the amounts of IgE are very small, even in highly atopic individuals, when compared with the levels of the other immunoglobulin classes. Consequently, background interference and the standardization of the system are difficult to arrange and much of the effort in laboratory investigation is directed to this area.

Methods of measurement of IgE and specific IgE antibody levels are well documented, but for a comprehensive and detailed review of basic methods readers are referred to Augustin (1975). Here we shall briefly summarize both the major methods of radioimmunoassay for IgE and some of the modifications which have been devised. More detailed discussion of the principles behind the various tests can be found in Chapters 4 and 5. As our work is mainly medical, most of the discussion in this chapter is about the measurement of human reaginic antibody, but much of the information is applicable to animals.

METHODS OF TOTAL IgE ESTIMATION

There are three radioimmunoassay methods available for the measurement of total IgE in a patient's serum (see Fig. 6.1) and several modifications of each method.

Competitive indirect assays (e.g. RIST)

The original method is a competitive, indirect assay (Johansson et al., 1968) in which the anti-IgE (usually raised in rabbits) is linked to an insoluble support such as cyanogen bromide-activated Sepharose (Wide et al., 1967). The patient's serum or a standard serum and a radiolabelled IgE preparation compete for attachment to the immobilized antiserum. After mixing and incubation the excess IgE (radiolabelled and unlabelled) is washed off and the amount of radioactivity in the precipitate is measured. The radioactivity remaining is inversely proportional to the amount of IgE in the patient's serum. The samples with standard serum dilutions, each of which has a known but different amount of IgE, are counted and the radioactivity is plotted against the IgE concentration. From this plot (graph or computer analysis) the amount of IgE in an

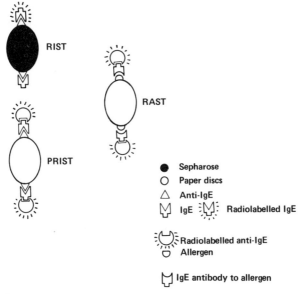

Figure 6.1. Diagram to illustrate the sequence of reactions
in RIST, RAST and PRIST assays

unknown serum can be accurately determined. The standard serum may be an IgE preparation diluted in IgE-free human serum or horse serum or it may be a serum from an atopic patient with a high IgE level. One improvement which can be made to this system (Nye *et al.*, 1975) is to pre-incubate the Sepharose/anti-IgE with the standard or patient's sera, adding the radioactive IgE as a second stage and after a second incubation washing as before. The pre-incubation allows more unlabelled IgE to attach, therefore allowing measurement of lower serum levels than would ordinarily be possible. Another modification (Catt and Tregear, 1967) is to couple the anti-IgE antiserum to plastic tubes rather than Sepharose as the insoluble phase, thus making the assay technically simpler.

Liquid-phase competition assays

A different method, which uses the competition principle, is the liquid-phase double antibody technique of Gleich *et al.* (1971). In this assay the IgE in the standard or patient's serum competes with radioactive IgE for attachment to (IgG) rabbit anti-human IgE; this complex is then precipitated by combination with a second antibody such as sheep or donkey anti-rabbit IgG. The radioactivity of the washed pellet is counted to measure the amount of labelled IgE bound and therefore the amount of IgE in the serum can be calculated by comparing the counts of the standard and unknown sera. A modification of this method of radioimmunoassay which has been used for measuring hormone levels is to pre-precipitate the second antibody or attach it to a solid phase (Brown *et al.*, 1980). This is said to allow a shorter incubation period and to improve sensitivity.

Solid-phase direct assays (e.g. PRIST)

More recent developments have led to the introduction of solid-phase direct methods for measurement of total IgE (Ceska and Lundkvist, 1972) (see Fig. 6.1). In these tests the anti-human IgE, usually raised in sheep, is linked to an insoluble phase such as cyanogen bromide-activated Sephadex, Sepharose or paper discs. The standard or patient's serum is allowed to react with the immobilized antiserum, then the unbound serum is washed off. Radioactive anti-IgE, usually raised in rabbits to minimize any cross-reaction of antisera, is added and after incubation attaches to the bound IgE. After the excess of radiolabelled antiserum has been washed off, the amount of IgE in the patient's serum can be measured by reference to the standard serum. This type of assay is technically simpler than either liquid-phase or solid-phase competitive assays.

Two solid-phase assay kits have been available from Pharmacia Ltd. for some years under the trade names Phadebas IgE Test (originally the Radioimmunosorbent Test, RIST) as the competitive assay and Phadebas IgE PRIST (Paper Radiommunosorbent Test) as the direct assay. The RIST-type assay, which has a higher working range than the PRIST is more sensitive for IgE levels below 50–60 μg ml (Johansson *et al.*, 1976; Merrett and Merrett, 1978a,b). At lower levels the RIST overestimates but the PRIST does not. The overestimation is probably due to protein fragments (not IgE) in the serum which link to the anti-IgE, thereby excluding the radioactive IgE and being measured as IgE molecules (Ceska and Lundkvist, 1972). In the PRIST assay these fragments which bind radioactive anti-IgE will not be measured unless they are divalent, as they are already bound to the immobilized anti-IgE. This effect is only seen with low levels of IgE when more radioactive IgE is bound in the indirect assay. In the PRIST assay there is an extra washing stage which allows immunoglobulin fragments and other serum proteins to be removed. Further, the PRIST assay is technically simpler and for these reasons it has tended to replace the RIST IgE test in routine use in most clinical laboratories. However, the RIST IgE test may still be used for accurate measurement of very high IgE levels when less dilution is needed than with the PRIST assay.

The liquid-phase assay is also available as a kit from Kallestad Ltd. (see Appendix) and in our experience is satisfactory, although it does require more technical expertise than the solid-phase assays using paper discs. The liquid-phase assay, however, has the advantage that it can be completed in a few hours without any loss in sensitivity compared with the overnight incubation necessary with the PRIST A fuller discussion on the use of commercial kits is given below.

METHODS FOR SPECIFIC IgE ANTIBODY ESTIMATION

From the earlier chapters it will have become obvious that measurement of total immunoglobulin levels is a poor substitute for *specific* immunoglobulin (antibody) assay, and so it is with IgE. The need to quantitate IgE specific antibody levels and to relate these to clinical phenomena is the important factor.

In this context an important development has been the introduction of assays of specific IgE antibody to a variety of allergens by the RAST technique. The basic method (see Fig. 6.1) is the direct RAST test (Radioallergosorbent Test) originally described by Wide *et al.* (1967), in which antigens are linked to an insoluble phase such as cyanogen bromide-activated Sephadex, Sepharose or paper discs. Specific IgE antibody from either a standard or patient's serum attaches to the antigen and, after washing to remove non-specific immuno-globulins and other proteins, the attached IgE antibody is detected by radiolabelled anti-human IgE (usually raised in rabbits and purified by affinity chromatography, prior to radiolabelling). The amount of antibody present is calculated by reference to a calibration graph obtained with a standard serum. The standard serum can be one which has a high antibody titre to the allergen in use, or one obtained by pooling a number of atopic sera and, under controlled conditions, it may be possible to relate the standard system to a different common allergen (see below).

Modifications of assays for specific IgE antibodies are variations on the basic RAST system as described above. One modification by Gleich *et al.* (1980) uses antigens linked to microcrystalline cellulose, which reduces the amounts of all the reagents needed. The assays to many allergens are as good as, if not better, than the basic technique. Another modification by Zeiss *et al.* (1973) is to coat plastic tubes with IgE and to link anti-IgE to the adsorbed IgE substrate. Test or standard serum is added in a second stage and IgE antibodies of all specificities will link to the anti-IgE. After removal of excess of serum proteins by washing, radioactive *antigens* are added and allowed to react during an incu-bation period. Further washing removes excess of radioactive antigen and the resulting radioactivity of the tube is then a measure of the specific IgE antibody in the serum. This method is very sensitive and the antibody can be quantified directly because the assay measures the primary binding of antigen and anti-body, as opposed to the secondary binding of antibody and antisera in the other RAST assays. However, pure proteinaceous antigens are required for this tech-nique and these are difficult to obtain. Further, when these are radiolabelled they are unstable, and there are therefore considerable technical disadvantages with the method.

The basic RAST assay has the advantage that relatively crude antigen prep-arations can be used and these have as long a shelf-life as the radiolabelled antisera.

An important aspect of the RAST assay is that underestimation of the amount of IgE antibody may occur in a sample containing large amounts of

IgG antibody (Kemeny *et al.*, 1980). The interference by IgG can be minimized by using a finely divided substrate or by having a large excess of antigen (Zimmermann *et al.*, 1980). It has been noted that low-avidity antibody is best detected when the antigen concentration is high and forms a stable bond with the substrate (Rubin, *et al.* 1980) and this may be an important factor in the assessment of IgE antibodies.

In recent years the RAST test has been available as a kit from Pharmacia Ltd. as Phadebas RAST. These kits cover a wide range of antigens although the list is not as comprehensive as those for skin testing. The antigens are linked to paper discs and are available either in lyophilized buffer or in moist buffered cassettes. The radiolabelled anti-IgE is raised in rabbits and is purified by affinity chromatography to be specific for the DE_2 antigenic determinant on the Fc fragment of human IgE. The reference reagents supplied with the kit are a set of birch pollen allergen discs and batches of diluted serum from a pool of human sera which have high IgE antibody to birch pollen (easily obtained in Sweden). Dilutions of the pooled sera are made in human serum which has no reaginic (i.e. IgE-mediated) activity to birch. The standardization of the reference system is linked to the Phadebas PRIST system, which in turn is linked to the International IgE standard (Lundkvist, 1975). In this way the company can maintain the accuracy of the system on a year-to-year basis despite changes of birch allergen and pooled reference sera. The use of one reference system for standardizing another can lead to difficulties. For example, a given level of binding of antibody to one allergen may not have the same clinical significance as the same binding to another allergen (e.g. the binding of antibody to moulds may be more significant than the same level of binding to commoner allergens). As with other immunoglobulin responses, the IgE response to a common allergen may be the result of exposure rather than clinical sensitivity and no clinical manifestations may be evident, even when a measurable amount of antibody is found.

GENERAL DISCUSSION

The use of kits

For the routine measurement of IgE, either total or specific, the use of a commercial kit must be considered. These kits are expensive but much of the expense can be offset against the time saved in preparing and purifying the antisera and antigens and in obtaining and purifying the standard sera, and also against the task of setting up and maintaining quality control of the whole system. Further, the use of kits makes less demand on the expertise of the laboratory staff, which may be an important point in small laboratories. If the technique is to be used for research these aspects may not be important, and there is then an advantage in using reagents made in the laboratory, i.e. in long-term studies the reagents are under the control of the researcher and can be varied at will as the work progresses. Further, commercial companies are continuously expanding the range of their reagents but this could cause problems if it occurred in the middle of a study. A compromise is to obtain commercially some of the reagents, especially those which are more difficult to prepare (e.g. radiolabelled antisera), and prepare the others in the laboratory. This is a common procedure, as a great deal of time can be spent preparing and purifying antisera to an antigen such as IgE, whereas allergens can be easily prepared.

Other methods for reducing the cost of kits are available. One method is to halve all the amounts of the reagents, including cutting the allergen discs in half. The halving of liquid reagents is simple but cutting the discs must be carried out with great care to ensure that each portion carries excess of antigen. Circular discs should be placed over lined paper to ensure that they are cut across the diameter. There is no problem with the discs in cassettes as these are hexagonal. The manufacturers do not recommend this, but we have used it successfully for RAST kits for several years. Several trials have been carried out and it has been found when comparing half and whole discs that there is agreement in 89% of all assays. With grass pollens, *Dermatophagoides pteronyssinus* and epithelia the agreement is about 90% and with foods about 84%. This compares well with the published figures for whole disc assays (Pharmacia Handbook on RAST). During one trial when a different panel of allergens and whole discs were used, a similar overall figure of 91% was obtained when the samples were assayed two or three times. These figures are admittedly lower than published values but most of the disagreement was found in the lower range of antibody levels (classes 1 and 2), and even here the absolute difference in the amount of antibody was not large.

Another factor is that of numbers; the accuracy of any procedure carried out manually on large numbers of specimens must lead to some lowering of performance when compared with assays of the same number carried out mechanically or of fewer numbers carried out manually. With the inherent errors of the system it is accurate enough for our purposes to use half-discs. One drawback to the use of RAST kits is that single estimations only for each patient are done for each antigen, and with large numbers of samples it is very easy for a mistake to be made. If a laboratory is considering using RAST kits and can afford to use whole discs, it is suggested that dual estimation on a patient's serum using half-amounts for each assay would be more worthwhile than single assays using whole discs. The PRIST kits are designed for the dual assay of each serum as is normal for most laboratory tests. Where liquid-phase assay kits are used (Kallestad total IgE) it is presumably possible that the amounts of these reagents could easily be halved, thereby lowering the costs of these kits. Further, liquid-phase assays are more easily adapted to mechanical processing than solid-phase assays. Some workers have suggested that some of the reagents may be re-used to reduce costs. Bruynzeel *et al.* (1978) suggested that the discs and unbound radiolabelled anti-IgE from RAST assays may be re-used, but such procedures should be monitored carefully and it may not be economical in view of the increased labour required and the decrease in accuracy.

There are two methods for reporting the results obtained with the Phadebas

94

RAST system. The most commonly used method is the RAST score, where the results of unknown sera are grouped in classes 0–4 by comparison with standard sera. The RAST test can, however, be calibrated in units similar to the PRIST test and the results of the unknown sera can be estimated with reference to the standard sera A–D in units/ml (see Appendix). We have always calculated the results in units/ml, although a general remark pertaining to the class of response is also made. This system is used because it enables the results to be documented more precisely, and is particularly valuable in follow-up studies. After desensitization therapy or during research projects it is useful to know the exact level of antibody not simply the RAST score. This is because the methods of calculation use a logarithmic scale, and there can be large differences between standards A, B and C within which there may be significant but 'invisible' changes of antibody level in the individual patient.

Total IgE *versus* IgE antibody measurement

An important question is whether it is necessary to estimate both total IgE and specific IgE antibody levels routinely in all patients. In our laboratories over the past 4 years 1818 patients have been screened for specific and total IgE. There was a difference in the correlation between the total IgE and specific IgE depending on whether the total IgE was measured by the RIST or PRIST test. The negative correlation was better using PRIST and the positive correlation better by RIST (Table 6.1). However, assuming the PRIST method to be more accurate, dual estimations carried out on about 800 specimens were examined, and it was found that 4% of patients have high total IgE (1000 units/ml), but normal RAST results; 23% of patients gave normal total IgE results but high RAST levels (i.e. one or more allergens of class 3/4 or more than three allergens of class 2). When moderately high levels are included, which may or may not be clinically significant, the combined figures are 30% and 42%, respectively (Table 6.1). It was also found that about 53% of all samples estimated for PRIST were high and 28% of the RAST were negative. It would appear from this that the RAST test would be the best preliminary assay. This is not the usual method of screening but it does not entail much extra work as judged by the numbers of positive PRIST tests which would need repeating for RAST and negative RAST that would need repeating for PRIST if all sera were double

Table 6.1. Relationship between total IgE levels (measured by PRIST) and specific IgE levels (measured by RAST)

	% High RAST	% Moderate RAST	% Normal RAST
% High PRIST	87.5	8.3	4.2
% Moderate PRIST	53.6	20.1	26.3
% Normal PRIST	22.8	19.0	58.1

checked. Any case histories sent with a sample should be studied and, if a clinician has noted a history strongly suggestive of atopy when the RAST screen is negative, a total IgE assay should then be performed. Such a policy allows the clinician to obtain useful information quickly, as high total IgE is not helpful compared with the results of specific antibody levels to various antigens which may indicate a causative allergen. This method of screening may be more expensive than initial screening of total IgE, but for the reasons outlined we believe that it is more satisfactory. The 'false negative' total IgE results can be explained by the fact that even if a patient is very allergic to one or two allergens the total IgE may not be raised.

A further argument for RAST screening in place of total IgE (by RIST or PRIST) measurement is that it will provide a baseline against which any changes during desensitization can be measured. It is important to define the antigen involved in atopy as well as the degree of immunological response.

However, even if it is decided not to screen using total IgE estimation, it must be remembered that some sera will require this investigation, particularly if the RAST results are difficult to interpret. Further, it is known that IgG_4 may sometimes be the cause of allergy, and in such patients the demonstration of a normal IgE level is important. There are numerous situations, not associated with allergy, where the patient's total IgE may be increased, such as parasitic infestations, myeloma, certain immunodeficiencies, e.g. Wiskott–Aldrich syndrome, thymic dysplasia and dermatological conditions, such as pemphigoid. It should also be noted that total IgE levels in childhood are well documented, whereas the expected specific IgE levels are not; young children (under 3 years old) have been found with very high RAST levels, usually to foods. It follows that total IgE levels have a definite place in diagnosis in children.

RAST and skin testing have been compared many times with different types of antigen (Wide and Juhlin, 1971; Berg and Johansson, 1974; Patrizzi et al., 1979). The results are all similar, and show good agreement (60–80%) between skin testing (using the prick test) and RAST. The agreement between provocation tests and RAST is slightly higher (90%), but in this case there is an increase in false-negative RAST.

There are other reasons for using RAST. Skin testing in the case of food allergies has been very unsuccessful and RAST results are definitely more reliable. Indeed, it could be argued that the RAST is the only relevant investigation in food allergy (Wraith et al., 1979). In dermatology clinics skin testing is not always suitable because many patients with hyperesponsive skin react even to negative control; here again RAST is invaluable. Skin testing is also difficult in children for practical reasons and RAST is often favoured. If the patient is very allergic there is a risk of a severe reaction to skin testing, and RAST is preferable. Finally, therapy with steroids and antihistamine drugs interferes with skin testing but these drugs have no known influence on RAST assays.

It is interesting that during the past 5 years the type of samples submitted to our laboratories has changed in composition as well as increasing four-fold in numbers. During 1977 and 1978 about 60% of the samples had very high total

IgE results (over 1000 units/ml) and about 15% of the samples were normal. During 1979 and 1980 these figures changed to 24% and 44%, respectively. Thus it would appear that since the test has become more widely publicized clinicians have become less selective in their submissions.

The allergen screen

If RAST tests are to be used for screening, a decision has to be made as to which allergens are to be included. Obviously, the maximum cover of allergens has to be reconciled with the cost of the tests and the literature recommends a minimum screen of three allergens; house dust mite (*Dermatophagoides pteronyssinus*), cat antigen and grass pollen antigen. In accordance with most published results it has been found in our laboratories that one or all of these three antigens is positive in 93% of atopic patients. Merrett and Merrett (1978a) have devised a three-in-one antigen for use in screening sera and identifying those which need more intensive study and they have reported good results. *D. pteronyssinus* antigen, grass pollen antigen and cat antigen are mixed together and linked to Sephadex particles. Under controlled conditions of antigen purity and reaction they claim results comparable to those with Phadebas RAST®.

We, however, routinely use a panel of seven allergens: *D. pteronyssinus*, cat, dog, grass pollens, milk, egg white and fish (cod). Of the last four allergens, dog and egg white are the most frequently positive, milk is next and fish is the least positive allergen.

We have found that the pattern of reactions is different for each antigen. Thus, house dust mite results in the 'high' classes (3 and 4) are present in 83% of cases, whereas class 2 responses are found in only 17%. The position is reversed with fish antigen, where 25% of cases have class 3 or 4 results, and 75% have class 2 results (see Fig. 6.2).

It should be noted that the above panel of antigens may be considered, by some, to be deficient. In particular, mould or fungal antigens and cereal antigens could be usefully included.

Our decision to extend the screening panel beyond the recommended three allergens can be justified by several facts. If house dust mite, grass or even cat allergens are found to be the agents responsible for an allergic response, they are not easily removed from the patient's environment. On the other hand, removal of food allergens is relatively easy and the demonstration of reaction to these is therefore important. Secondly, many infants and young babies are screened in our laboratories and recent work has indicated that the development of atopy in later life may be signalled by abnormal IgE levels (total and specific) in infancy. A complete screen in these children is therefore of considerable value. After testing 200 children under 5 years of age, it was found that the pattern of sensitivity was very different from that of adults in that specific IgE antibodies to food allergens were more common; this has also been noted by other workers (Bjorksten and Johansson, 1975). In our study it was found that children under 1 year of age reacted most strongly to egg white, milk, grass pollen

% in different classes

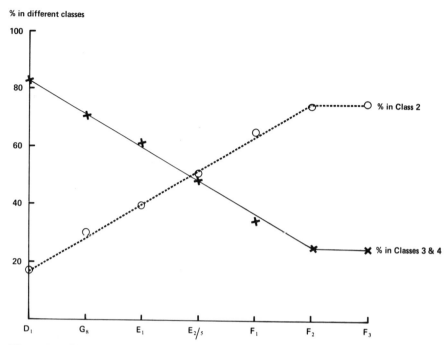

Figure 6.2. Diagram to show the incidence of high- and low-grade reactions to different allergens. The allergens used were: D_1, *D. pteronyssinus*; E_1, cat; F_1, egg white; F_3, codfish; G_8 grass pollen; $E_{2/5}$ dog; F_2 cows' milk

and fish, and least to *D. pteronyssinus*. It is often mentioned in the literature that children under 1 year of age do not develop allergy to pollens because they have not lived through two pollen seasons. We have found a few young children (under 1 year) who have antibody to grasses, and although this may seem to be at variance with other reports it can be explained by the fact that they were all about 1 year old, and had probably been exposed to the end of one pollen season and the beginning of the next. In younger babies the levels of antibody to grass were lower and may have a reflected some cross-reaction with pollens from other sources (e.g. cereals in the diet). In the age group 1–2 years, egg white was the allergen which caused most responses. In the final group, aged 2–5 years, *D. pteronyssinus* was the allergen which caused most responses but dog allergen and egg white were still common. Reaction to pollens was not as common as in the adult. By the age of 9 years the adult pattern of antibodies was established. Therefore, if screening procedures are required for children's samples, food allergens are important. However, it seems that food sensitivities in children are often outgrown and may not present clinical problems in later life.

Most of the samples from children received in our laboratories come from those aged under 1 year and over 11 years, and this probably reflects the use of the test by the clinician as a screen in early months and later as problems arise near puberty.

We have included dog allergens in the screening panel because the dog is a common family pet. There are two available allergens, dog epithelium and dog dander. The former allergen was used in a clinical study (Mackie et al., 1979) and positive results were found to correspond well with the contact a patient had with dogs. This is in contrast to the cat allergy, which does not seem to provoke responses related to the amount of animal contact. It would seem that the cat allergen is either a potent antigen producing large amounts of antibody after minimal contact or it cross-reacts with a common antigen in the environment. In a recent study, Merrett and Merrett (1979) compared dog dander and dog epithelium antigens, and suggested that dog epithelia produced more false-negative results, but they noted that dog dander allergens cross-react with antibodies to cat or horse antigens in about 25% of patients, these being patients with allergy to cats or horses but not dogs. They recommend care in the interpretation of results with dog dander but prefer its use to dog epithelium. Both antigens have been used in our laboratories and it has been found that the number of positive results to dog epithelium and dander was almost the same (about 23%). There was, however, a slight shift in the range of response, in that more results in classes 3 and 4 occurred with dog dander (53%) than with dog epithelium (44%). Other work (Valito et al., 1980) has demonstrated that the allergenicity can vary significantly between different batches of dog dander preparations from both the same manufacturer and different manufacturers. All of this emphasizes the importance of adequate quality control of antigen preparations, and the need to assess each batch against a standard serum of known potency. This is particularly important if the allergen preparations are prepared in the laboratory.

Another point to consider when using either laboratory preparations or commercial kits is the cross-reaction between different grass pollens. Several grass pollens were used in our laboratories for about one year. No differences in reaction were found in any patient to the different grasses, i.e. if the patient was positive to one, he was positive to all. Other work (Leiferman and Gleich, 1976) has shown that there is extensive cross-reaction between many of the common grasses, with Timothy, Bermuda and Sweet Vernal grass pollens being slightly different from the others. The best policy would seem to be to choose a common local grass, with the exception of the three mentioned. With ragweed pollen antigens (a common source of allergen in the USA) work has been done (Leiferman et al., 1976) which has shown that there is extensive cross-reaction between different types, with Slender and Southern ragweed, however, being less active than the Giant and Western varieties. With extracted and purified antigens from ragweed pollen Adolphson et al. (1978) found that AgE was more commonly allergenic than the other four major antigens of the pollen. There was substantial cross-reaction between AgE and AgK but less between antigens Ra_3, Ra_4 and Ra_5. This again emphasizes the need for strict quality control of the assay and careful choice of the antigens.

Also of interest when investigating seasonal allergy is that moulds can be potent antigens. It has been shown in hay fever in the USA that moulds such as Alternaria may be at least as important as common pollens such as ragweed (Feinberg, 1936).

It is worth noting that we do not use house dust preparations in our laboratories because we have considered that the major antigen of house dust is the house dust mite and, although other allergens may be involved, these will probably be peculiar to the patient's own home, e.g. animal danders of various pets. For this reason it does not seem to us to be worth testing a 'standardised' house dust. Other workers (Pauli *et al.*, 1979) have confirmed the complex nature of house dust sensitivity, and supported this concept.

Finally, it should be mentioned that much has been done to control the quality of antigens for allergy tests. Many patients are skin tested as well as RAST tested, especially in research projects, and in these circumstances it is helpful if the antigens are as pure as possible for both tests to enable the results to be correlated. The quality of skin testing antigens are to some extent regulated by health and safety regulations, but allergens for RAST may be of any quality.

It is obviously difficult to use the same antigens in both skin tests and RAST assays, for these reasons, but there is a good case for 'assessing' skin tests in accordance with their RAST reactivity. This can be done by establishing the amount of inhibition produced by different skin test allergens in RAST assays of different patients. In this way it is possible to bring each set of allergens into line and this may allow more useful comparisons between the results of each type of test. Control of this kind is even more important in the preparation of vaccines, because clearly it is necessary to include those antigens which are responsible for the patient's hypersensitivity and to exclude irrelevant materials. It will be of interest to see whether industry, which has done so much to assist the diagnosis and management of allergy, will respond to this challenge.

A further reason for ensuring maximum purity of allergens is that in long-term studies the results must be comparable and this means that variation must be minimal. If the antigen is pure it is easier to standardize the assay. Schroeder and Yman (1980) mentioned that when a large pool of high titre sera is used, a representative sample of all the different specificities of antibody will be present. Using such a sample they compared batches of antigen of different ages and found, perhaps surprisingly, good agreement between the results. However, with kits it is important to have minimal batch variation, because antibodies to one antigen are compared with those against another (the standard system being birch pollen antigen and sera with high anti-birch IgE antibody).

The most common method for checking the quality of an antigen preparation is the inhibition of RAST assays (see above) in which solid-phase and liquid-phase allergens compete for antibody in sera. The amount of inhibition of binding to the immobilized allergen by the standard liquid-phase antigen is related to the purity of the bound allergen. Huggins *et al.* (1980) have developed a method for standardization of the RAST against the WHO standard IgE preparation, which relates inhibition of different preparations to absolute units of IgE antibody absorbed from the test sera. This method is independent of antigen preparation, source of atopic sera and other variables. Other methods of RAST inhibition were given in more detail by Aalberse (1980).

The use of total IgE estimations

There has been renewed interest in levels of IgE in the very young, because it has been known for some years (Kjellman, 1976) that in children under 1 year of age, 75% of those who have a total IgE level above + 1 S.D. from the normal develop atopic disease, compared with only 6.4% of children with levels below the + 1 S.D. value. Other workers (Soothill et al., 1976) have shown that children who have one or two allergic parents commonly have positive skin tests in the first year of life and that these reaginic manifestations are related to presymptomatic, transient IgA deficiency. In these studies the RAST or total IgE levels were not helpful, but there have been refinements of the techniques since then. It has been suggested by Soothill (1976) that in some genetically predisposed children the IgA system is immature and during the period when low levels of IgA exist, exposure to antigens can allow IgE antibodies to develop. Other investigators (Kemp, 1979; Bjorksten et al., 1980) have shown that children born during times of high seasonal levels of antigen have an increased incidence of positive skin tests to these antigens. The possible danger of 'feeding' allergens to susceptible infants has been emphasized by Soothill (1976), who has suggested that feeding with synthetic or cows' milk may allow abnormal gut flora to develop and this, coupled with low IgA levels, may permit antigens to cross the intestinal mucosa and initiate IgE responses in these predisposed babies. If this hypothesis is correct, breast feeding during the first year of life should decrease the amount of IgE produced during the period of IgA maturation. Saarinan et al. (1979) demonstrated that infants fed with breast milk did have lower IgE levels than infants fed with cows' milk and that this was not due to the presence of specific antibodies to cows' milk. There is no evidence, however, to suggest that the substitution of soy milk for cows' milk is beneficial in the suppression of atopic symptoms in children up to 4 years of age (Kjellman and Johansson, 1979). As a result of this kind of work, it seems probable that the measurement of total and specific IgE antibodies in children will become more important in screening and also in further research. In some recent work it seems (Yates, personal communication) that specific IgE antibodies may be useful in predicting which type of infantile dermatitis is atopic in origin.

Food allergy and RIA

There is a need for further investigation of food allergy in adults. Diagnosis of food allergy is particularly complex because reactions may be either food intolerance where there is no IgE antibody involvement or true food allergy associated with abnormal IgE response. Furthermore, reactions to foods may occur immediately after ingestion of the food or up to several hours later, making the diagnosis difficult. Another difficulty is that the allergen may be a breakdown product of the food rather than the food itself, and this complicates the preparation of pure, insoluble antigens. Recently, the allergic response and intolerance of certain people to food additives such as azo dyes and preservatives has been studied, and August (1980) has suggested that the use of food additives linked to albumen in RAST assays may be useful in the study of these reactions.

Further, other studies have attempted to investigate the link between the occurrence of IgE antibodies to food and the development of diseases which are not obviously atopic, e.g. migraine (Monro et al., 1980). It is accepted, however, that more work is needed on the purification of food allergens for both RAST assays and skin testing because a significant number of non-specific reactions do occur. When pure food allergens are available it may be possible to examine more closely the links between food allergy and other atopic manifestations, e.g. urticaria and eczema.

Measurement of IgG4

Another area of interest related to total and specific IgE estimation is the measurement of the other reaginic antibody, IgG_4. This has been shown to have important reaginic activity particularly in eczema and RAST-type assays of IgG_4 antibodies and radioimmunoassays for total IgG_4 level are becoming more common. Preliminary work by Bruynzeel and Berrens (1979) would seem to indicate that some antigens stimulate IgE antibodies rather than IgG_4 whilst others stimulate both classes of immunoglobulin equally. It is possible, therefore, that the total reaginic response and the response against specific allergens will in future be measured with reference to both IgE and IgG_4. There are no commercial kits yet available for the measurement of IgG_4 but the basic principles of preparing the reagents are as outlined above. The amounts of immunoglobulin in subclasses of antibody are as small or smaller than those of IgE type and there will inevitably be problems of sensitivity in developing these assays. However, this is an area which must be developed in the future.

CONCLUSIONS

It will be clear that whilst there are certain indications for the use of radioimmunoassay of IgE antibody (see p. 95), there are many other instances which could be regarded as 'research' areas, where the use of the method is not validated but may offer promise. In our view, any deficiencies in the diagnostic use of RAST and similar assays arise from inadequate investigation. This view is based on the fact that IgE antibody is the heart of the allergic problem and to measure, monitor and assess this response is fundamentally important. However, we are aware that other parts of the immune response can significantly 'modify' the effect of IgE antibody. Notably, IgG (of subclasses 1, 2 and 3) antibody may fulfil its classical role as a 'blocking' antibody, rendering the IgE incapable of activating the mast cells and producing symptoms.

The importance of this to the investigator is that it would be wise to measure both IgE and IgG antibody to particular antigens. There is no reason why this should not be done. Much of this book has been devoted to a discussion of methods of measurement of IgG antibody to various antigens, and it must only be a matter of time before the measurement of IgG antibody to 'allergens' becomes routine. The assay of IgG for allergens is particularly important for monitoring patients during desensitization therapy, because it is clear that a good response to the latter may occur for either of two reasons. In some patients the specific IgE antibody disappears very quickly, and these individuals need no further desensitization treatment. In others, the specific IgE level remains high but IgG antibody increases and 'blocks' the hypersensitivity reaction. These patients probably require regular booster injections of antigen to maintain the IgG response. Thus, it would seem important to elaborate the *type* of response to desensitization, and this in our view can only be achieved by simultaneous assay of IgG and IgE antibody levels. It is interesting that Pharmacia Ltd., the manufacturers of the Phadebas RAST® kits, have recently introduced one such 'dual' kit, which can measure IgE and IgG antibody to insect venoms. The introduction of other more varied developments offers an exciting and, we believe, rewarding prospect for the management of allergy.

REFERENCES

Aalberse, R. C. (1980). IgE based radioimmunoassay for the quantitation of allergens. *Allergy*, **35**, 236–238.

Adolphson, C., Goodfriend, L., and Gleich, G. S. (1978). Reactivity of ragweed allergens with IgE antibodies. *J. Allergy Clin. Immunol.*, **62**, 197–210.

August, P. J. (1980) in *Proceedings of First Food Allergy Workshop*. Medical Educational Services, Oxford, pp. 76–81.

Augustin, R. (1975). Techniques for the study and assay of reagins in allergic subjects, in *Handbook of Experimental Immunology* (Ed. D. M. Weir). 3rd ed., Vol. III. Blackwell Scientific Publications, Oxford, pp. 451–456.

Berg, T. L. O., and Johansson, S. G. O. (1974). Allergy diagnosis with the radioallergosorbent test. *J. Allergy Clin. Immunol.*, **54**, 209–221.

Bjorksten, F., and Johansson, S. G. O. (1975). *In vitro* diagnosis of atopic allergy. *Clin. Allergy*, **5**, 363–373.

Bjorksten, F., Suoniemi, I., and Koski, V. (1980). Neonatal birch-pollen extract and subsequent allergy to birch-pollen. *Clin. Allergy*, **10**, 585–591.

Brown, T. R., Bagchi, N., Ho, T. T. S., and Mack, R. E. (1980). Pre-precipitated and solid-phase second antibody compared in radioimmunoassay. *Clin. Chem.*, **26**, 503–507.

Bruynzeel, P. L. B., Van den Bogaard, W., and Berrens, L. (1978). Re-utilization of I^{125}-labelled anti-IgE antibody and paper discs in PRIST and RAST IgE determination. *Clin. Chim. Acta*, **90**, 297–300.

Bruynzeel, P. L. B., and Berrens, L. (1979). IgE and IgG_4 antibodies in specific human allergies. *Int. Arch. Allergy Appl. Immunol.*, **58**, 344–350.

Catt, K., and Tregear, G. W. (1967). Solid-phase radioimmunoassay in antibody coated tubes. *Science*, **158**, 1570–1571.

Ceska, M., and Lundkvist, U. (1972). A new simple radioimmunoassay method for determination of IgE. *Immunochemistry*, **9**, 1021–1030.

Feinberg, F. M. (1936). Seasonal hay fever and asthma due to moulds. *J. Am. Med. Assoc.*, **107**, 1861–1867.

Gleich, G. J., Averbeck, A. K., and Swedlund, H. A. (1971). Measurement of IgE in normal and allergenic serum by radioimmunoassay. *J. Lab. Clin. Med.*, **77**, 690–698.

Gleich, G. J., Adolphson, C. R., and Yunginger, J. W. (1980). The mini-RAST compared with other varieties of RAST for measurement of IgE. *J. Allergy Clin. Immunol.*, **65**, 20–28.

Huggins, K. G., Roitt, I. M., Brostoff, J., and Taylor, W. A. (1980). Standardisation of radioallergosorbent test and allergen extracts in terms of the W.H.O. Standard for IgE. *Allergy*, **35**, 224–226.

Johansson, S. G. O., Bennich, H., and Wide, L. (1968). A new class of immunoglobulin in human serum. *Immunology*, **14**, 265–272.

Johansson, S. G. O., Berglund, A., and Kjellman, N. I. M. (1976). Comparison of IgE values as determined by different solid-phase RIA methods. *Clin. Allergy*, **6**, 91–98.

Kemeny, D. M., Lessof, M. H., and Trull, A. K. (1980). IgE and IgG antibodies to bee venom as measured by a modification of the RAST method. *Clin. Allergy*, **10**, 413–421.

Kemp, A. S. (1979). Relationship between the time of birth and the development of immediate hypersensitivity to grass pollen antigens. *Med. J. Aust.*, **1**, 263–264.

Kjellman, N. I. M. (1976). Predictive value of high IgE levels in children. *Acta Paediatr. Scand.*, **65**, 465–471.

Kjellman, N. I. M., and Johansson, S. G. O. (1979). Soy versus cows milk in infants with biparental history of atopic disease. Development of atopic disease and IgE from birth to four years of age. *Clin. Allergy*, **9**, 347–358.

Leiferman, K. M., and Gleich, G. J. (1976). The cross reactivity of IgE antibodies with pollen allergens I. *J. Allergy Clin. Immunol.*, **58**, 129–139.

Leiferman, K. M., Gleich, G. J., and Jones, R. T. (1976). The cross reactivity of IgE antibodies with pollen allergens. II. *J. Allergy Clin. Immunol.*, **58**, 140–148.

Lundkvist, U. (1975). Research and development of RAST technology, in *Proceedings of 1st N. American Conference on RAST* (Ed. R. Evans). Symposia Specialists, Miami, pp. 85–101.

Mackie, R. M., Cobb, S. J., Cochran, R. E. I., and Thomson, J. (1979). Total and specific IgE levels in patients with atopic dermatitis. *Clin. Exp. Dermatol.* **4**, 187–195.

Merrett, J., and Merrett, T. G. (1978a). RAST atopy screen. *Clin. Allergy*, **8**, 235–240.

Merrett, T. G., and Merrett, J. (1978b). Methods of quantitation of circulating IgE. *Clin. Allergy.*, **8**, 543–557.

Merrett, T. G., and Merrett, J. (1979). Epithelium or dandruff allergen for the diagnosis of dog allergy by RAST. *Clin. Allergy*, **9**, 429–435.

Monro, J., Brostoff, J., Carini, C., and Zilkha, K. (1980). Food allergy in migraine. *Lancet*, **2**, 1–4.

Nye, L., Merrett, T. G., London, J., and White, R. J. (1975). A detailed investigation of circulating IgE levels in the normal population. *Clin. Allergy*, **5**, 13–24.

Patrizzi, R., Muller, U., Yman, L., and Hoigne, R. (1979). Comparison of skin tests and RAST for the diagnosis of bee sting allergy. *Allergy*, **34**, 249–256.

Pauli, G., Bessot, J. G., and Thierry, R. (1979). Inhibition experiments with solid-phase mite or epithelia in house dust hypersensitivity. *Allergy*, **34**, 311–318.

Rubin, R. L., Hardtke, M. A., and Carr, R. I. (1980). The effect of high antigen density in solid-phase radioimmunoassay for antibody regardless of immunoglobulin class. *J. Immunol. Methods*, **33**, 277–292.

Saarinen, V. M., Bjorksten, F., Knekl, P., and Siimes, M. A. (1979). Serum IgE in healthy infants fed breast milk or cows milk-based formulas. *Clin. Allergy*, **9**, 339–345.

Schroeder, H., and Yman, L. (1980). Standardisation of RAST inhibition assay. *Allergy*, **35**, 234–236.

Soothill, J. S. (1976). Some intrinsic and extrinsic factors predisposing to allergy. *Proc. Roy. Soc. Med.*, **69**, 439–442.

Soothill, J. S., Stokes, C. R., Turner, M. W., Norman, A. P., and Taylor, B. (1976). Predisposing factors and the development of reaginic allergy in infancy. *Clin. Allergy*, **6**, 305–319.

Valito, T., Viander, M., and Koinkko, A. (1980). Skin-prick tests in the diagnosis of dog dander allergy: comparison of different extracts with clinical history, provocation tests and RAST. *Clin. Allergy*, **10**, 121–132.

Wide, L., Axen, R., and Porath, J. (1967). Radioimmunosorbent assay for proteins. Chemical couplings of antibodies to insoluble dextran. *Immunochemistry*, **4**, 381–386.

Wide, L., and Juhlin, L. (1971). Detection of penicillin allergy of immediate type by radioimmunoassay of reagin (IgE) to penicilloyl conjugates. *Clin. Allergy*, **1**, 171–177.

Wraith, D. G., Merrett, J., Roth, A., Yman, L., and Merrett, T. G. (1979). Recognition of food-allergic patients and their allergens by the RAST technique and clinical investigation. *Clin. Allergy*, **9**, 25–36.

Zeiss, C. R., Pruzansky, J. J., Patterson, R., and Roberts, H. (1973). A solid phase radioimmunoassay for the quantitation of human reaginic antibody against ragweed antigen E. *J. Immunol.*, **110**, 414–421.

Zimmermann, E. H., Junginger, J. W., and Gleich, G. J. (1980) Interference in ragweed pollen and honey-bee venom RAST tests. *J. Allergy Clin. Immunol.*, **66**, 386–393.

Chapter 7

Clinical use of radioimmunoassay of antibody

GENERAL COMMENTS

The aim in this chapter is to illustrate how radioimmunoassay of antibody can be used in patient care, whether from the view of the laboratory worker or the clinician. One of the important attributes of radioimmunoassay, which was alluded to in Chapter 1, is its ability to define in detail the antibody response of a patient. Most diagnosticians are familiar with the general principles of serological analysis by conventional methods, i.e. recognition of rising titres after infection or falling titres much later, but the detail which RIA can provide is new to most people and requires to be understood. We have chosen in this chapter to use certain diseases as examples in an attempt to show the value of the method in the management of the patient. The diseases discussed are those with which we have most experience, and are not to be considered as exclusive examples.

EXTRINSIC ALLERGIC ALVEOLITIS

The term allergic alveolitis is a general one which includes many conditions, all caused by a hypersensitivity reaction in the lungs to inhaled antigens. The lung is diseased because antigen and antibody combine in the alveoli, stimulate an Arthus-type hypersensitivity and lead ultimately to pulmonary fibrosis. Some of the best known examples are farmer's lung, pigeon breeders' disease, maltworkers' disease and humidifier fever. A full list of these conditions can be found in Pepys (1969).

The diagnosis of these conditions has been difficult in the past, but Pepys *et al.* (1963) and Pepys and Jenkins (1965) showed that patients with farmers' lung often have precipitins to antigens which are present in mouldy hay and which are derived from an actinomycete, *Micropolyspora faeni*. Precipitins are simply detected by allowing the antigens and the patient's serum to interact in a gel. All that one can establish from such a test is that the patient has antibody to the antigens, and this can only indicate that the patient has been exposed to these antigens and has responded to them. Early reports indicated that this simple test was useful in diagnosis, but several groups later reported that patients with typical symptomatology and histories were negative by this test (Jameson 1968; Grant *et al.*, 1972). Further, there were many patients who had precipitins but were symptomless.

These seemingly paradoxical results were resolved by the use of radio-immunoassay (Parratt *et al.*, 1975) of antibody to the antigens of *M. faeni*. In Fig. 7.1 the distribution of antibody levels in this disease is shown for a mixed group of normals, symptomless farmers and symptomatic farmers. There is a spectrum of levels, from the low responses of urban dwellers to the very high responses of the most seriously affected farmers. If the clinical status is added (Fig. 7.2) it can be seen that whilst normals tend to be below a level of 30 μg/ml, and severely affected individuals above 80 μg/ml, between these levels there is a mixture of symptomatic and symptom-free farmers and the antibody level *per se* cannot be diagnostic. In short, the antibody level cannot be regarded as diagnostic, and by extension of the argument it cannot either be diagnostic at the low or high points of the scale. What is clear, though, is that there is a *greater probability* of disease at the high end of the scale, and a *lesser probability* at the lower end. It is important to recognize that this interpretation, which is biologically sound, has only been possible by looking at *many* patients, whereas the diagnostician usually only has one patient to work with. This, then, is the first benefit of RIA. Because of its sensitivity and accuracy it has shown the true pattern of antibody responses in the population and has indicated that reliance on a single antibody measurement is bound to be inaccurate on occasions. It may seem, at first, a negative finding, but it should not be regarded so because it indicates, by greater description, the true picture and at the same time shows that an alternative to diagnosis in the individual patient is required.

A better approach is to study changes of antibody level. In infections, one assumes (see Chapter 1) that a new exposure to the infecting organism will lead to an increase of antibody, and whilst this may happen in farmers' lung it is confused by the fact that many patients will have antibody because of long exposure to small amounts of antigen. In short, an increase may not be easily detectable, even with the sensitivity of the RIA method. However, this disease is caused by combination of antigen and antibody in the lungs and the onset of disease should therefore be associated with a decrease in serum antibody levels. Indeed this is so, as shown in Fig. 7.3 (see also Fig. 1.6), but the difficulty is that unless the patient has been recently reviewed and unless he presents early after the onset of symptoms, such a decrease in antibody is unlikely to be observed, and again the diagnosis must be circumstantial. It is doubtful whether antibody measurement in these diseases can ever provide proof of the diagnosis, although it can support the diagnosis. The latter must remain essentially clinical, and in these diseases clinical interpretation can be very difficult.

It is clear from the results of RIA analysis that antibody can be accurately and sensitively quantitated. It is also clear that without antibody the disease

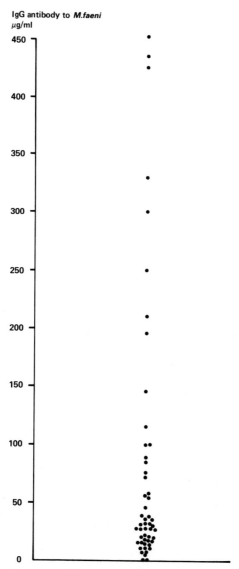

Figure 7.1. The distribution of levels for 54 sera assayed for IgG antibody to *M. faeni*. The sera include farmers with a history of symptoms, healthy farmers and healthy urban dwellers. The need for an assay which works over a wide range is clear

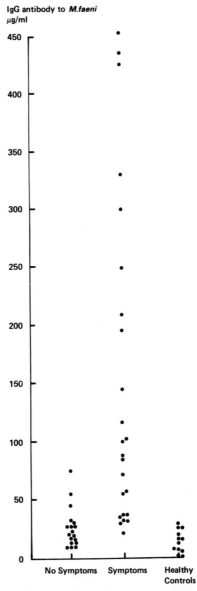

Figure 7.2. The distribution of IgG antibody levels to *M. faeni* in symptomatic farmers, asymptomatic farmers and healthy urban controls

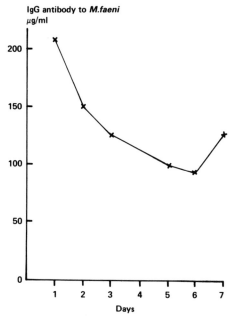

Figure 7.3. The fall in IgG antibody (to
M. faeni) in the few days following an acute
episode of farmers' lung. Towards the end of
the period of study the antibody level was
beginning to increase

will not occur, and by projection it is likely that antibody will not be produced if
exposure to antigen is prevented. Therefore, if antibody levels are monitored,
evidence can be obtained which will indicate the degree to which an individual
has been exposed to antigen. The results of a study of this type are shown in
Table 7.1, where the summer and winter antibody levels of several patients are
compared. Summer levels would be expected to be low in this disease because
the cattle are grazing outdoors, whereas in winter they are fed indoors with
mouldy foodstuffs. As shown in Table 7.1, some individuals do respond by
producing antibody in the winter but others do not, and this simple test will
therefore indicate those who are being progessively exposed to mouldy
materials. Prevention of this exposure will prevent the disease occurring.

   In farmers' lung, therefore, RIA has not radically improved the laboratory
diagnosis in the sense that it will confirm or refute the diagnosis absolutely.
What it has done is to illustrate the background biology, or at least humoral
immunity, of the disease, and has shown how prevention of the disease may be
achieved.

   Full technical details of the farmers' lung RIA were given by Parratt *et al*.
(1975), but some of these details are relevant to general discussion.

   Firstly, for routine assay of samples it is advisable to quantitate over a wide

110

Table 7.1. Comparison of summer (August) and winter
(March) levels of IgG antibody to *M. faeni* in 13 farmers

Patient	Summer level (μg/ml)	Winter level (μg/ml)	Change (%)
1	27.2	46.0	+69.1
2	71.3	44.0	−38.3
3	436.2	407.1	−6.7
4	21.3	29.6	+38.9
5	36.3	55.1	+51.8
6	35.3	51.5	+45.9
7	38.0	34.5	−9.2
8	17.2	24.0	+39.5
9	76.2	49.0	−35.7
10	21.3	29.6	+38.9
11	188.7	210.5	+11.5
12	116.2	103.0	−11.4
13	210.5	470.0	+123.3

range of levels, in order to reduce the number of repeat tests. Inevitably, to accommodate the samples with the highest levels of antibody the amount of antigen supplied to each sample must be large to provide the necessary excess of antigen for antibody binding (see Chapter 5).

For most samples the amount of antigen will be excessive, and the assay is therefore wasteful, but this is not a serious problem because it is easy to culture large amounts of *M. faeni*. This may not be the case with some antigens, and in such cases it will be necessary to limit the range of the assay, accepting that very high level samples and possibly low level samples may need to be re-assayed. However, it is usual in diagnostic work to identify a level below which the sample is considered as 'normal' and not therefore requiring accurate measurement.

A further point to note is that the assay, across its wide range, quantitates to an accuracy of within 5–10%. It has been argued that such an accuracy is not required for diagnostic purposes but, if we accept that monitoring of the level in the individual patient is necessary (see above), the antibody level must be measured accurately on each occasion. It is easier to do this if the accuracy of routine assays is maintained, otherwise the alternative is to treat each set of serial samples as 'special cases', with different assays for different patients.

A final question is whether the RIA of antibody in farmers' lung is the best way of measuring the antibody. Early work (see above) showed that the method was superior to the precipitin test which is commonly used for diagnosis. In view of the fact that the precipitin test is as effective as agglutination, haemagglutination and complement fixation tests, it follows that RIA is the best method for analysis of antibody. Recently, an ELISA (enzyme-linked) assay was described (Barndad, 1980). Broadly, the results were similar to those with RIA obtained many years earlier, but the accuracy and therefore the differentiation appear to be inferior at low and moderate levels of antibody. This may be because the parameter which is finally measured is absorbance, which cannot be measured as accurately as the radioactivity of a sample. Against this it must be added that the ELISA technique was superior to the precipitin test. The question is for each investigator to decide the method he or she is to use, according to the sensitivity required and the methods available.

The discussion above has concentrated on farmers' lung but the principles apply in the other diseases of similar type.

BRUCELLOSIS

This disease presents an interesting problem for the diagnostician. In most cases, isolation of the organism is not possible, or at least is not achieved, and the diagnosis depends on serological methods. In some cases serodiagnosis by conventional means is straightforward, in that it is possible to demonstrate an increase in antibody titre by agglutination of the organism, in a simple tube dilution procedure. Further, by carrying out a Coombs-type test (that is, washing the organisms from the first agglutination test and adding some anti-human immunoglobulin) it is possible to establish whether IgG (incomplete and poor at agglutination) antibody is present in the sample. It is customary, therefore, to regard a high titre in the direct agglutination test as indicative of early, acute infection, and a high titre in the indirect test as that of a more chronic infection. A complement fixation test is also available and is said to be particularly valuable in chronic cases of the disease.

The use of RIA which measured IgG, IgM and IgA antibody to *Brucella abortus* indicated that there was no close correlation with the standard tests, except between IgG estimation and the indirect agglutination test (Parratt *et al.*, 1977). There were cases, very illuminating, where other evidence of brucellosis was strong and where RIA detected antibody which was not shown by agglutination or complement fixation tests. These, together with the poor correlation between results, indicates that reliance on 'biological activity' of antibody may sometimes lead to a false result, because some antibodies will not agglutinate or fix complement and cannot be detected by measuring these activities. The question remains as to whether the standard tests should be abandoned and replaced by RIA. Where facilities exist, this is probably the ideal, but in other centres it may be better to continue the use of the standard tests and refer difficult specimens to a reference laboratory which can perform RIA. Thus, any sample which is negative by the ordinary methods when the patient gives a history suggestive of brucellosis should be referred. Any sample which is from a patient with continuing illness should also be referred because frequent monitoring is necessary in chronic cases, and this is best done by RIA.

CANDIDA ALBICANS ANTIBODY ASSAY

Many methods for measuring antibody to *C. albicans* have been described and were reviewed by Axelson (1976). Most of the methods are conventional procedures for the detection of antibody and depend on precipitation, agglutination or complement fixation. These tests have been developed to diagnose deep-seated *C. albicans* infections. In most cases they have been only partially successful for reasons which have become clear only with the use of radioimmunoassay of antibody (Cobb and Parratt, 1978). Using the RIA method (see Fig. 7.4) a healthy population are found to have widely differing levels of serum antibody to *C. albicans*. Further, as is the case in farmers' lung (see above), the conventional precipitin test becomes positive only at high levels (70 μg/ml IgG antibody), and is therefore positive only in a minority of cases. This would be satisfactory if there was always a large increase in antibody in those people who were infected with the organism, but two lines of investigation show that this is not always so.

Firstly, patients with serious infection are certain to have large numbers of organisms in their body, and these organisms will absorb antibody and lead to a fall in the circulating level of antibody. This can be shown by studies of the most severe infection of all, candidaemia, a representative example of which is depicted in Fig. 7.5. It is clear that antibody is undetectable at the time of candidaemia, but increases rapidly in the period after resolution of the infection. Thus, in those most severely ill, it is likely that antibody levels will remain low and therefore undetectable by crude tests such as precipitin tests. This problem is made worse by the fact that many patients who contract *C. albicans* infection are immunosuppressed and have low antibody responses at the outset.

Secondly, it is clear from studies of patients who are particularly susceptible to candidaemia, such as those in intensive therapy units, that colonization by Candida and an antibody response to the organism is common (Fig. 1.7). This

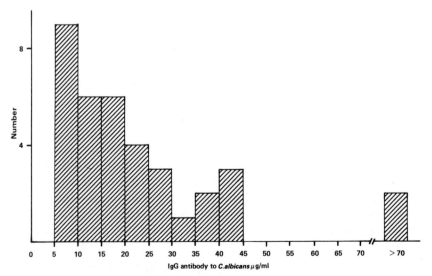

Figure 7.4. Distribution of serum IgG antibody levels to *C. albicans* in 35 healthy donors. (Reproduced by kind permission of the *Journal of Clinical Pathology*)

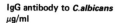

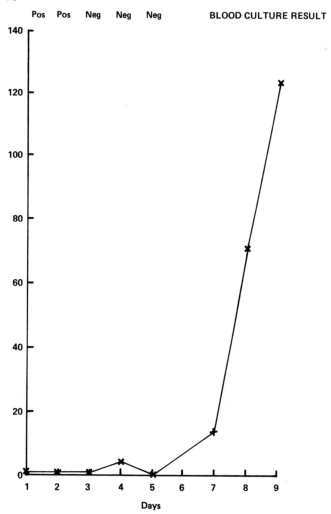

Figure 7.5. A study of serum IgG antibody levels to *C. albicans*
during and after candidaemia (proved by blood culture)

colonization probably arises because the patients are receiving 'prophylactic' antibiotic therapy. Certainly, the effect of antibiotic therapy on colonization by *C. albicans* and antibody response to the organism is easily demonstrated and can be shown by simple experiments on normal persons, who receive a small amount of antibiotic over a short period of time (see Figs. 7.6 and 7.7).

The results given in Figs. 7.6 and 7.7 point to another important advantage of quantitating antibody during short periods. Fig. 7.6 shows the changes of antibody before, during and after a short course of oral tetracycline therapy (Ig.

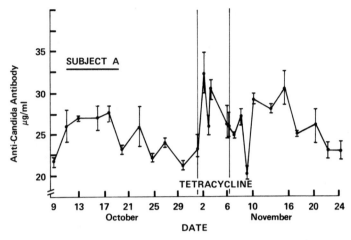

Figure 7.6. Results of a study of IgG antibody levels to *C. albicans* in a healthy individual, before, during and after tetracycline therapy. The error bars indicate the variation between triplicate samples. Some errors are large and the values cannot be regarded as significant, but most samplings have low errors

daily for 5 days). The changes are small, when one considers that the range for normal persons is 0–60 μg/ml, and do not appear to form a particular pattern. However, this analysis is crude in that it does not take time into account. If the data are replotted as *change* of antibody relative to time (i.e. rate) the results are more meaningful. It is clear that the antibody production rate is in equilibrium before the tetracycline therapy, responds very quickly during the therapy and thereafter settles to the basic rate. Although the absolute levels of antibody do increase during the therapy, they are not markedly elevated and the change is

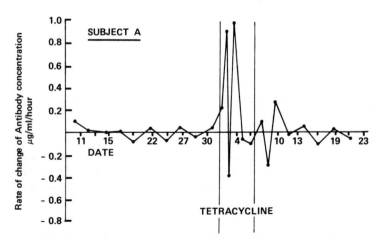

Figure 7.7. The results shown in Fig. 7.6 plotted as rate of change of IgG antibody to *C. albicans* (μg/ml/h)

best shown by observing the rate of change of antibody level. Longer courses of tetracycline, however, do cause much larger increases than shown in this example. It should be clear, though, that the changes of level are so delicate and rapid as to require a very sensitive and accurate assay for their detection.

It should be noted that the increase in colonization and the parallel increase of antibody level in patients in intensive care does not lead to infection in most cases, and the finding of high antibody levels does not necessarily have diagnostic significance. As in the case of farmers' lung, the measurement of antibody to *C. albicans* by RIA adds a new dimension to serological analysis, allowing the response to be analysed in terms of its biology. The RIA permits a detailed monitoring of the events before, during and after any incursion by this organism, and in this respect outlines the true course of infection rather than providing a firm (or assumed) diagnosis of infection. It must be noted, though, that it does not resolve the diagnostic problem, and only highlights the deficiencies of the existing methods of investigation. It follows from the findings shown in Fig. 1.7 that an increase of antibody means only that the patient has been colonized and the result itself has no diagnostic significance. This is a radical departure from the concepts of classical microbiology, where (as indicated in Chapter 1) it is held that an increase of antibody to a microorganism is considered to indicate a recent infection. The difference is that the classical approach was developed for organisms which were uncommon, i.e. organisms producing epidemic disease, whereas *C. albicans* is a commensal organism which is normally found in the body and which occasionally produces infection. There are many organisms like *C. albicans* which cause infections, and the dynamics of their populations and the antibody responses to them are probably similar.

The discussion above has indicated many of the problems which face the modern serologist. The question which must be asked is, how can a true infection be diagnosed?

It seems likely that serious infection is associated with a *fall* in antibody level and it may therefore be relevant to monitor the levels of antibody and suspect problems when such a decrease occurs. This idea is admittedly contrary to all the traditional serological views, but is nevertheless logical and offers a new way out of a difficult dilemma. A further important development is to assay immune complexes, which are the product of antigen and antibody interaction, and have a unique status in the interpretation of host–parasite relationships. The possibilities for such investigations, as yet relatively unexplored, are discussed below in the section on immune complex radioimmunoassay.

In summary, it cannot be said that RIA of antibody to *C. albicans* has improved the *diagnosis* of infection by this organism. What it has done is to improve the understanding of the balance which normally exists between this organism and the host and has indicated the directions in which further work must proceed. It is a good example of the fine line between research and diagnostic usage and emphasizes the fact that good diagnosis ultimately depends on adequate research and that the latter must include the most detailed appraisal possible. In studies of the antibody response to *C. albicans* this is clearly the case.

IMMUNE COMPLEX ASSAYS

There are many immune complex assays which are not radioimmunoassays and therefore have no relevance in this book. The interested reader will find references and comparative data in a WHO-sponsored study (Lambert *et al.*, 1978), where information on radioimmunoassays is also available.

Before discussing the available assays it is worth noting the importance of immune complex estimation in clinical work. There are many diseases which are thought to be caused by immune complexes, or to be exacerbated by them. The former group are often referred to loosely as the 'connective tissue diseases' and include rheumatoid arthritis, polyarteritis, polymyositis, systemic lupus erythrematosis and Sjögren's syndrome. In addition, acute glomerulonephritis and serum sickness are well known and well established examples of immune complex diseases.

In these examples the disease is usually widespread in the body but in some conditions such as extrinsic allergic alveolitis (see above) the damage is localized to one organ. It is possible and it has been frequently suggested that some disorders of the intestine and gut, such as ulcerative colitis and Crohn's disease, may also be immune complex diseases, although it is more likely that these fall into the second category of conditions where immune complexes form secondarily to the primary disease and cause an exacerbation of the condition. It can be argued (see below) that in all infections a similar exacerbation of symptoms due to immune complexes may occur.

Immune complexes produce damage by lodging in the tissues and fixing complement. This produces chemotactic factors for polymorphonuclear leucocytes and these, when they arrive at the site of activation, cause damage to the tissues by releasing their enzymes. The damage caused is healed by fibrosis, and the long-term effects of all immune complex diseases are loss of structure and function after fibrosis. The severity of the ensuing disease is related to the amount of complex formed and the length of time for which these complexes persist. For this reason it is essential that the investigation of immune complex diseases includes accurate assay of the complexes which are causing the damage to the tissues. This is becoming particularly relevant because plasmapheresis and drug therapy can now reduce the level of complexes. There is one, important, proviso which is that the assays available measure immune complexes in serum (or plasma) and therefore may not reflect the processes which are occurring in the tissues. This argument is compelling and cannot, as yet, be answered easily. Basically it is sound theoretical reasoning, although even in those conditions where localized disease is present (e.g. farmers' lung) there is evidence of generalized involvement if one looks for it. Therefore, serum immune complex measurement may be valuable. Further, it is established that in some 'localized' infections such as chronic otitis media generalized immune complex manifestations such as glomerulorephitis sometimes occur. Whether these assays will prove to be of clinical value in these conditions is questionable, but the matter can be resolved only by performing assays by the most sensitive methods, and radioimmunoassays must be included amongst these.

Immune complexes will be produced in any instance where antibody is raised against a soluble antigen and this includes most immune responses. It is particularly true of infections. Fig. 1.4 indicates that from the beginning of infection the organism grows and increases its population, and during this time will shed antigens so that the antigen content will also increase. At the same time antibody is forming and the interaction will produce immune complexes.

In the early part of the infection the complexes have a large excess of antigen, but with time they become slight antigen excess complexes and are finally formed in antibody excess.

At all points in this course immune complexes will be present, in varying amounts, and these will contain the antigen or antigens which are derived from the microorganism. These should be detectable by appropriate methods, and if detected will identify the responsible microorganism. The advantage of following this course of investigation is that it may be possible to establish a diagnosis at a much earlier point in the infection than cultural or conventional serological methods can achieve. Particularly, it is likely that at the onset of symptoms, or even before this, the most effective method of diagnosis would be recognition of the immune complexes and the identification of their antigenic component.

Perhaps the real value of immune complex assays will, in the future, lie not so much in their detection, but in their description. The ability to identify the antigenic component will add to the diagnostic precision in the 'immune complex diseases' and at the same time provide new opportunities for rapid diagnosis in other conditions.

In the past immune complexes have been associated with generalized autoimmune disease, particularly systemic lupus erythematosus. As indicated above, there are other diseases outside the autoimmune conditions in which immune complex damage is important. However, it will be clear from the account below of radioimmunoassays of immune complexes that some have been developed solely to investigate immune complex disorders. Some assays for auto-antibodies are also mentioned below.

RADIOIMMUNOASSAYS OF IMMUNE COMPLEXES

Rheumatoid Factor assays

One of the principles used in the assay of immune complexes is inhibition or competition by rheumatoid factor for immune complexes. Rheumatoid factor is a 19S (IgM) antibody found in the serum of patients with rheumatoid arthritis which reacts with 7S (IgG) immunoglobulin, particularly when the latter is structurally modified. In some cases it is possible to observe, and isolate, monoclonal rheumatoid factor (RF) from the serum, and where this is possible the RF can be used as a reagent for immune complex assays. The RF is coupled to cellulose (see Chapter 2) and reacted with iodinated aggregated human IgG, which it will bind efficiently. If similar reaction mixtures are set up which contain immune complexes, the latter will compete with the aggregated IgG for binding to the RF. Thus a reduction of bound isotope indicates the presence of immune complexes, and the amount of reduction in radioactivity will quantitate the level of these complexes. Aggregated IgG is frequently used in immune complex assays as a substitute for immune complexes. Whether this is valid is not clear, but with the present state of the technology it is the simplest and therefore most widely used alternative. IgG prepared immunochemically is aggregated by heat at 63 °C for 30 min and quantitated by spectrophotometry or immunochemical methods.

The RF assay, which is very sensitive, is not interfered with by the presence of polyclonal rhematoid factor in the test sample and has been found to correlate with the severity of disease symptoms. While the assay requires purified monoclonal rheumatoid factor, only very small amounts are needed per test (approximately 2 μg bound to 27 μg of cellulose). The major disadvantages of the method are that it is essential to analyse each sample initially by radial immunodiffusion for monomeric IgG content and the monoclonal rheumatoid factor required is not readily available. There are several variants of the above principle which have been developed to avoid some of these technical difficulties, but it should be noted that up to 40% of all sera tested may be unassayable because of autoagglutination of the reagents by the test samples (see Lambert *et al.*, 1978).

Clq assays

Immune complexes may also be detected and quantified by the Clq binding test. Clq is the first component of complement and as such it binds to antibodies which are attached to antigen. Clq is separated by chemical methods (Yonemasu and Stroud, 1971) and radiolabelled (by the lactoperoxidase method, Chapter 3) and the test relies on the binding of radiolabelled Clq to immune complexes in a test sample. After suitable incubation, unbound Clq is removed by addition of sheep erythrocytes sensitized with IgG antibody (an antigen–antibody system) in the absence of complement. The liquid phase may then be enumerated for retained radioactivity separately from the cell phase. A variation is to use polyethylene glycol at a concentration of 7.5% to precipitate the immune complexes. In this way, the radioactivity bound to the complexes is precipitated also, and after removal of the supernatant the radioactivity can be measured, as representative of the amount of immune complex in the test sample. Alternatively, Clq may be attached to a solid phase (see Chapter 2) reacted with the test serum and binding detected by a labelled anti-globulin reagent. These tests are technically simple to perform but have the disadvantages that purified Clq is required, and that they only measure immune complexes containing antibody which can fix Clq. Another disadvantage of the Clq binding test is that Clq can bind non-specifically to DNA and lipopolysaccharide, resulting in false-positive tests.

C3 binding assays

A further RIA technique for measuring immune complexes is the Raji cell binding test. Human lymphoblastoid cells (Raji) which are transformed cell lines (by Epstein–Barr virus) have on their surface receptors for the third component of complement (C3) and one of its fragments C3c. Immune complexes which have bound complement display C3c and can attach to the surface of the cells. After attachment they may be detected using an iodinated antiglobulin reagent which is added after thorough washing of the cells. The technique has several disadvantages. Firstly, it depends on complement fixation by the complex. Secondly, Raji cells also react with antibodies which have auto- or allo-specificity for cellular components, and this is a problem which can be overcome only by blocking the reactive sites with suitable immunoglobulin fragments. However, this makes the test difficult to perform in many laboratories. Thirdly, the maintenance, standardization and monitoring of Raji cells for the presence of complement receptors is tedious, and requires considerable expertise in the laboratory.

It is worth noting that the importance of complement fixation by immune complexes is a difficult question. On the one hand, it is possible to argue that only those complexes which can fix complement will be important as a cause of tissue damage and, therefore, that the method chosen should rely on detection of complement-containing complexes. On the other hand, it is reasonable to argue the reverse, that non-complement-fixing complexes have some biological activity. This question will be resolved only by careful studies using techniques which will detect one or other, or both, types of immune complex.

Another RIA for immune complexes is based on their ability to bind to conglutinin. This assay is similar to the Raji cell assay in that conglutinin also binds to C3c. Conglutinin is a non-immunoglobulin protein which to date has been described only in members of the family Bovidae. Domestic cattle are the most convenient source of the substance. The ability to bind fixed C3c may be utilized in assays by attaching conglutinin to a fixed matrix such as plastic tubes, beads or Sepharose®, removing unbound material be washing and then reacting the product with the test specimen. If C3c-bearing immune complexes are present, these will bind to the conglutinin and, after washing, they can be detected by the addition of a radiolabelled antiglobulin reagent.

The conglutinin assay is technically simple to perform; the only purified material needed being conglutinin which is relatively easy to prepare from bovine serum by absorption with zymosan and pepsin digestion (Maire et al., 1981). It does have certain disadvantages, however, such as the need for conglutinin titration before selection of a bovine serum for its purification because conglutinin levels vary considerably in different animals. A variation of the procedure is similar to the C1q assay described above in that isolated and radiolabelled conglutinin is mixed with the test sample and any complexes present are thereafter precipitated with polyethylene glycol and the radioactivity is measured.

Although all of the above assays have certain disadvantages, the use of radioactive tracers have made them more sensitive for detecting fluid-phase immune complexes. There are, however, a number of reports in the literature describing discrepancies in the results obtained when the same sera are assayed with various tests. These differences may arise because the properties of the tests are variable, as indicated above. Alternatively, it may simply be that small soluble immune complexes, able to bind to C1q or monomeric rheumatoid factor, are unable to bind C3 components. This would make them undetectable by Raji cells or conglutinin. Whatever the reasons before the meaning of these tests both in a research and in a diagnostic setting can be established, these discrepancies must be understood.

An assay has been described which is a novel combination of biological and radioimmunoassay principles (Mohammed *et al.*, 1977). Guinea pig macrophages have binding sites for Fc, and therefore will absorb radiolabelled aggregated globulins, if reacted with these. The addition of immune complexes will interfere with the absorption and the decrease in binding of radiolabelled globulin is proportional to the amount of complex added. Thus the method is very similar to a competitive binding assay for antigen, except that living cells are the substrate for the attachment of the reactants. The difficulty with this assay is that of obtaining the macrophages and preserving them in a state which ensures maximum efficiency in the test. For some laboratories this will be relatively easy, but in other cases it may prove to be difficult.

In the above discussion reference has been made to the use of polyethylene glycol to precipitate immune complexes. A simplified technique using this property for the measurement of IgG–anti-IgG immune complexes in rheumatoid arthritis has been devised. In this method radiolabelled IgG interacts with anti-IgG (rheumatoid factor) and forms immune complexes which can be precipitated with polyethylene glycol. Such simple techniques, which do not rely on any secondary interactions, are useful. Other assays including some for the detection of immune complexes to viral agents have been developed using polyethylene glycol. Evidently, polyethylene glycol does not precipitate uncomplexed IgG.

Finally, it is worth remembering that the assay chosen for measurement of immune complexes depends on whether the investigator wishes to detect the antigenic component of the complex or whether he is interested only in the level of circulating complexes. As a generality the C1q and RF binding assays are difficult to adapt to antigen determination. The Raji cell and conglutinin assays, on the other hand, will easily perform this function and it is possible with polyethylene glycol precipitation assays, if the precipitated complex is dissociated and the antigen component identified.

Radioimmunoassay of auto-antibodies

Rheumatoid factor (RF), a 19S (gM) antibody which reacts with 7S (IgG) immunoglobulin, is a constant, and important feature in the serum of patients with rheumatoid arthritis. It is now known that RF can exist in a 7S (IgG) form. Traditionally, RF has been detected by agglutination of particles (sheep red cells or latex) which are coated with IgG. A radioimmunoassay which uses rabbit immunoglobulin bound to plastic tubes has been described, in which RF attaches to the rabbit Ig and is, after washing, detected by applying a radiolabelled anti-globulin (either anti-IgM or anti-IgG). Another assay measures antinuclear antibody. Antinuclear antibody occurs in the serum of patients with systemic lupus erythematosus and was initially detected by the LE cell test and by an indirect immunofluorescence test. However, RIA procedures have been developed using either cellular antigens or purified deoxyriboncleic acid (usually derived from calf thymus and commercially available). In most of these assays, the antigen is insolubilized by linkage to plastic beads or tissue culture tubes (see Chapter 2). Antibody to the DNA is detected by a conventional solid-phase assay as described in Chapter 5. Alternatively, antinuclear antibodies may be measured in a liquid-phase assay using radiolabelled DNA as the antigen (Chapter 4).

Antibody to acetylcholine receptor can also be measured by RIA. Lindstrom *et al.* (1976) found that 91 of 93 sera from patients with myasthenia gravis contained antibody to acetylcholine receptor.

REFERENCES

Axelson, N. H. (1976). Analysis of human Candida precipitins by quantitative immunoelectrophoresis. *Scand. J. Immunol.*, **5**, 177–190.

Barndad, S. (1980). Enzyme-linked immunosorbent assay (ELISA) for IgG antibodies in farmer's lung disease. *Clin. Allergy*, **10**, 161–171.

Cobb, S. J., and Parratt, D. (1978). Determination of antibody levels to *Candida albicans* in healthy and hospitalised adults using a radioimmunoassay. *J. Clin. Pathol.*, **31**, 1161–1166.

Grant, I. W. B., Blyth, W., Wardrop, V. E., Gordon, R. M., Pearson, J. C. G., and Mair, A. (1972). Prevalence of farmer's lung in Scotland: A pilot study. *Br. Med. J.*, **1**, 530–534.

Jameson, J. E. (1968). Rapid and sensitive precipitin test for the diagnosis of farmer's lung using immuno-osmophoresis. *J. Clin. Pathol.*, **21**, 376–382.

Lambert, P. H., *et al.* (1978). A W.H.O. collaborative study for the evaluation of eighteen methods for detecting immune complexes in serum. *J. Clin. Lab. Immunol.*, **1**, 1–15.

Lindstrom, J. M., Einarson, B. L., Lennon, V. A., and Seybold, M. E. (1976). Immunogenicity of syngeneic muscle acetylcholine receptor and quantitative extraction of receptor and antibody–receptor complexes from muscles of rats with experimental auto-immune myasthenia gravis. *J. Exp. Med.*, **144**, 726–738.

Maire, M. A., Barnet, M., and Lambert, P. H. (1981). Purification of bovine conglutinin using pepsin digestion. *Mol. Immunol.*, **18**, 85–89.

Mohammed, I., Thompson, B., and Holborow, E. J. (1977). Radiobioassay for immune complexes using macrophages. *Ann. Rheum. Dis.*, **36**, 49–57.

Parratt, D., Nielsen, K. H., Boyd, G., and White, R. G. (1975). The quantitation of antibody in farmer's lung syndrome using a radioimmunoassay. *Clin. Exp. Immunol.*, **20**, 217–225.

Parratt, D., Nielsen, K. H., White, R. G., and Payne, D.I.H. (1977). Radioimmunoassay of IgM, IgG and IgA brucella antibodies. *Lancet*, **1**, 1075–1078.

Pepys, J. (1969). Hypersensitivity diseases of the lung due to fungi and organic dusts. *Monogr. Allergy*, vol. 4.

Pepys, J. and Jenkins, P. A. (1965). Precipitin (FLH) test in farmer's lung. *Thorax*, **20**, 21–35.

Pepys, J., Jenkins, P. A., Festenstein, G. N., Gregory, P. H., Lacey, M., and Skinner, F. A. (1963). Farmer's lung: thermophilic actinomycetes as a source of 'farmer's lung hay' antigen. *Lancet*, **2**, 607–609.

Yonemasu, K., and Stroud, R. M. (1971). Cl_q: rapid purification method for preparation of monospecific antisera and for biochemical studies. *J. Immunol.*, **106**, 304.

Chapter 8

Further application of radioimmunoassay to the study of antibody

INTRODUCTION

Radioimmunoassay (RIA) of antibody should have its influence in two broad areas, viz. (1) development, with automation, for diagnostic purposes and (2) application to specialized investigations of the basic knowledge of immunology. Its application to the latter is important but has often been ignored. Immunology has tended to develop using long-established techniques of antibody assessment and has only recently resorted to the more flexible and informative primary binding assays such as RIA. This chapter will deal with RIA as applied to research, including those procedures developed for diagnosis, and will be largely composed of contributions selected from the literature. It will consider the detection and quantitation of antibody to:

Human viruses and viral antigens

Bacteria and bacterial antigens

Other infectious agents and small molecules

Immunoglobulins, autoantibodies, idio- and allotype antibodies

Tumour antigens

Experimentally used antigens

Drugs

In addition, the general advantages of RIA over other primary binding assays and secondary methods of estimating antibody will be discussed in the context of these topics with various modifications of RIA. This is not intended to be a complete review of the literature, but an indication of the applicability of RIA as a research method. Therefore *selected* reports from the literature will be considered in detail.

Finally, we must add that the range of assays considered is wide and we do not have personal experience in all of these areas. The style of this chapter is therefore different from the foregoing, the reader being referred to literature reports rather than our own experiences.

VIRUSES AND VIRAL ANTIGENS

The human viruses most commonly studied by RIA are herpes simplex virus, hepatitis B virus and rubella virus. RIA techniques for measurement of antibody to these do not vary greatly and fall into two basic categories: (1) liquid-phase assays and (2) solid-matrix assays.

Liquid-phase assays

There are two basic types of liquid phase assay. Firstly, a radiolabelled virus may be used either by itself or in a competition assay with unlabelled virus for binding sites on immunoglobulin molecules, which are contained in a prepared antiserum to the particular virus. The immune complexes formed between the antigen (mixture) and antibody may be removed from unreacted antigen by precipitation either with a chemical such as ammonium sulphate (provided that 'free' virus is soluble in sulphate), as in the Farr assay, or by addition of an antiglobulin reagent (see Chapter 4). The precipitate formed is removed by centrifugation, washed and enumerated for radioactivity. When labelled virus is mixed with serum-containing antibody, a higher radioactive count in the precipitate indicates greater amounts of antibody. If a mixture of labelled and unlabelled virus is used the results are more difficult to interpret. Thus, if a measured amount of labelled antigen is used with an excess of unlabelled antigen, a low count would indicate a high antibody binding capacity of the serum. Conversely, if a measured amount of unlabelled virus is used with an excess of radioactive virus, a high count would indicate large amounts of antibody. The latter type of assay would obviously be more difficult to perform.

The second type of liquid-phase RIA for virus includes the reaction of viral antigen with antibody (serum) and then removal and washing of immune complexes by centrifugation. This requires a high-speed centrifuge as the primary complexes are small. Antibody bound in the complex may then be measured by the addition of radiolabelled antiglobulin. This is a modification of direct RIA (see Chapter 5). The secondarily formed immune complexes are again removed and washed by centrifugation and enumerated for radioactivity. A high count indicates a large amount of antibody in the complex, the amount of contained radioactivity being directly proportional to the amount of antibody present. The removal of unwanted reagents at all steps in the above three procedures can be carried out by filtration of complexes on appropriately equilibrated mini-columns of Sephadex which are chosen to exclude complexes and retain unbound materials. The difficulty with the technique is that it cannot be applied to a large number of samples, although a modification using gel filtration *and* centrifugation to remove unattached reactants has been described by Fránek and Hruska (1976), and this may extend the usefulness of the method in diagnosis.

Solid-phase assays

Several RIAs using a solid matrix have been described but they have one feature in common, namely that the antigen (virus) is immobilized by attachment to a particulate substance. The particulate substance varies depending on the properties of the virus. Thus, rubella and herpes simplex virus have been attached to filter-paper discs, microtitre plates [poly(vinyl chloride)] and polystyrene balls (Kalimo et al., 1977). The mechanism of attachment is poorly understood but may include van der Waals forces, which presumably may lead to non-specific binding of other protiens, in turn leading to unwanted cross-reactions. Other coupling agents for the immobilization of viruses are m-diazobenzyl-oxymethylene cellulose for hepatitis virus (Duimel and Brummelhuis, 1975), polypropylene tubes for hepatitis virus (Ling and Overby, 1972), monolayers of influenza-infected cell lines (Schieble and Cottam, 1977), glass cover-slips for vaccinia and herpes virus (Hutchinson and Ziegler, 1972) and polystyrene tubes for myxovirus and vaccinia virus.

The concensus from the literature suggests that plastic microtitre plates are the most useful because most antigens will bind to them, and a large number of samples can be handled if the test is automated. It should be noted, however, that the choice of a matrix is important for each virus–antibody system because it is influenced by virus attachment, and by the elimination of non-specifically bound proteins.

In these assays, the matrix-bound virus is incubated with antibody (serum), washed and then incubated with a radiolabelled antiglobulin reagent (see Chapter 5). This is followed by further washing and then enumeration for retained radioactivity. The higher the isotope count, the larger is the amount of antibody. One of the advantages of this system is that the washing procedures are simpler if a solid-phase assay is used. For example, polystyrene balls can be manipulated with forceps, and washing machines are available for the microtitre system. Microtitre plates, however, cannot be counted for radioactivity as easily as polystyrene tubes or balls because the plate must be dismembered prior to counting in conventional gamma/scintillation machines. As an alternative, a special device capable of counting the intact plate can be used.

OTHER INFECTIOUS AGENTS AND SMALL MOLECULES

RIA methods for the detection of antibody to yeasts, moulds, actinomycetes and parasites are described in the literature. These do not vary from those described above (and Chapter 5) and to avoid repetition will not be described in detail. Similarly, RIA for drugs, chemicals and hormones have been reviewed by Skelley et al. (1973) and Butler (1975), and will therefore not be included, because these are essentially assays of 'antigen', not antibody.

IMMUNOGLOBULINS, IDIOTYPES AND ALLOTYPES, AND OTHER BODY FLUID SUBSTANCES

A variety of techniques are available for the measurement of total immunoglobulin levels of a given class or subclass in body fluids. Immunoglobulins are to be regarded as any other serum protein and the measurement of these is not strictly assay of 'antibody', although clearly the immunoglobulins are constituted by antibodies of many specificities. For completeness this section is included, although the reader should keep in mind that antibody activity in these assays is not being measured.

Most assays of immunoglobulin rely on precipitation with an appropriate antiserum and include immunoelectrophoresis, quantitative double and radial immunodiffusion and electroimmunodiffusion. They are subject to considerable error, and are relatively insensitive, making the measurement of small amounts of immunoglobulin difficult. The development of RIA primary binding methods for immunoglobulin levels has increased the sensitivity of these estimations, and has found a particular place for those immunoglobulins which are present in small amounts. A good example is that of IgE in serum (Chapter 6), but the situation is often similar for other immunoglobulins in body secretions.

Immunoglobulins

Solid-phase assays

The primary binding assay techniques in general rely on the insolubilization of anti-heavy chain IgG molecules to a matrix, such as Sephadex® (Wilde, 1969), Biogel (Nerenberg and Prasad, 1975) or plastic (Catt, et al., 1966). Polyvinyls have been shown to be the most useful of the latter (Herrmann and Collins, 1976). The matrix-bound antibody is incubated with the fluid (to be measured), washed and reacted with the *same* anti-heavy chain IgG preparation, which in the second stage is radioactively labelled. After washing, the retained radioactivity is counted and the value obtained gives a direct measurement of the amount of immunoglobulin present.

This type of method uses the same anti-heavy chain preparations on either side of the 'sandwich', and this reduces interference by cross-reacting substances present in the sera. The technique is also highly specific because an anti-heavy chain antiserum of high specificity is used, which eliminates competitive interference by other immunoglobulin classes. Since both the sensitivity and specificity are high, small amounts of immunoglobulins in fluids may be measured accurately. Nerenberg and Prasad (1975) reported measurements of as little as 25 ng per 100 μl of IgA and 10 ng per 100 μl of IgM in cerebrospinal fluid with this type of assay.

As is the case with other RIA methods, calibration graphs using positive samples of known immunoglobulin concentrations or highly purified immunoglobulin preparations of known weight are essential for accurate measurement. This is not, however, a disadvantage as myeloma proteins of all the human and most animal immunoglobulin classes are available. Nevertheless, to obtain accurate and reliable results, the molecular binding capacity of both the matrix-bound and the labelled anti-heavy chain preparations must exceed the content of the immunoglobulin in the fluid to be measured. Consequently, it is usually necessary to test the serum at a 10-fold dilution in addition to the neat concentration or, alternatively at two greater dilutions, which are apart by a factor of 10.

Liquid-phase assays

Liquid-phase competition RIAs may be used with a standard amount of radiolabelled antigen (immunoglobulin) preparation, but this requires double (antibody) anti-immunoglobulin precipitation. Assays such as these have been described (Beeken and Roessner, 1975), but have been tedious and extravagant in terms of purified antigen (Chapters 4 and 5 deal with the principles of the above methods).

Two novel methods for measuring IgE immunoglobulin also exist. One is based on the fact that IgE which is antibody bound is insoluble in 33% ammonium sulphate, whilst unbound IgE is soluble. In this method radiolabelled IgE can be used in a liquid-phase competition assay to measure IgE levels (see Farr test—Chapter 4). The second method uses radiolabelled Fab′ anti-IgE antibody which, after reaction with IgE, can be removed as an immune complex by precipitation with 45% ammonium sulphate. Unbound Fab′ is not precipitated at this concentration, and this method is more sensitive than the 'sandwich' technique, the PRIST method and previously described assays for IgE (Chapter 6). A disadvantage is the difficulty of preparing Fab′ fragments of IgG anti-IgE.

Allo- and idiotypes

RIA has proved useful in the study of allo- and idiotypes of immunoglobulin molecules. A double antibody ('sandwich') RIA procedure has been used to measure the human allotype $Gm(b^0)$ on IgG_3 molecules. The method consists of preparing an anti-allotype antibody of the required specificity by absorption of unwanted reactivity. This is attached to a solid matrix and using the same antiserum, radiolabelled, the concentration of the particular allotype can be measured in a test sample. Similarly, allotype determinants of the V_H and light chains of rabbit IgG and IgA have been investigated by a modified ammonium sulphate precipitation method. A liquid-phase RIA for the determination of chicken 7S immunoglobulin–heavy chain allotypes has been employed, and a solid-phase (plastic tube) RIA for the investigation of mouse immunoglobulin allotypes has been described. In addition, V_H determinants associated with rabbit T-lymphocytes have been investigated by RIA and human myeloma protein idiotypes have been studied by a 'sandwich' RIA procedure. Although all of these studies have required the absorption of antisera to make them specific for the genetic determinant(s) under study, the adaptation of the RIA procedure has greatly increased the sensitivity of detection of these determinants, and it is likely that this type of RIA, particularly the liquid-phase competition assays, have a future in allotype and idiotype investigations. Also, RIA should prove useful in the study of dissociated immunoglobulin domains and for the detection of small mediator molecules such as lymphokines. No radioimmunoassays for lymphokines have been reported (to the authors' knowledge), but such a procedure, using highly specific antibody, would be preferable to current assays employing cell functions, such as macrophage migration inhibition or transfer of delayed hypersensitivity.

The difficulty in this area is that of producing antibody to the lymphokines. From a purely practical point of view, the most important stimulus for antibody production is to provide easy and reliable assays for transfer factor. This substance may or may not be a true lymphokine but even if it is not accepted as such it typifies the problems in this area. Transfer factor is obtained from lymphocytes as a small peptide (molecular weight less than 12,000) which can transfer delayed hypersensitivity from donor to recipient. It has an impressive record in some diseases where cellular immunity is depressed, but the major difficulty is that having prepared the material there is no simple method of determining how much active material is present. Many workers use the material without any check of activity, whilst others perform laborious tests which involve measuring its activity against cultured cell lines, or in intact animals. Antibody to transfer factor can, however, be produced using either an alum-adsorbed preparation which is injected into rabbits regularly over many months, or by coupling the material to a carrier protein prior to immunization in a conventional way (see Chapter 3). It is not yet certain that the prepared antibodies are wholly satisfactory, or that their specificity is of the required type, but the fact that antibodies have been raised makes it likely that radioimmunoassay of this material will be possible soon.

Other serum substances

Although perhaps not directly within the scope of this book, it would be inconsistent not to point out the versatility of RIA procedures by illustrating their use in the detection and measurement of body fluid substances other than immunoglobulins. Since this is not an all-inclusive review of the literature, only a few will be included. These are:

Procollagen (Taubman et al., 1974)
B2 microglobulin (Plesner et al., 1975; Vincent and Revillard, 1976; Taniguchi et al., 1976).
α-Fetoprotein (Forrester et al., 1975)
Lactoferrin (Bennet and Mohla, 1976)
Ferritin (Luxton et al., 1977)
C-reactive protein (Claus et al., 1976)
α-Lactalbumin (Kleinberg, 1975)
Hemopexin, albumin and haptoglobin (Kida and Muller-Eberhard, 1975)
Hageman factor (Saito et al., 1976)
Melatonin (Arendt et al., 1975)

Antibody to tumour antigens

Some of the earliest applications of RIA of antibody were in tumour immunology. Tanigaki et al. (1966) used radiolabelled antisera (heavy chain specific) to detect immunoglobulin biosynthesis by human leukaemia cells *in vitro*. Similarly, Harder and McKhann (1968) demonstrated absorption of mouse antibody directed against normal H-2 antigen on normal lymphoid cells and sarcoma cells using a radiolabelled anti-mouse globulin reagent. Ting and Herberman (1971), on the other hand, used an isotope-labelled antiglobulin to detect antibody to polyoma tumour cell surface antigens. Reif (1971) modified the technique by using a paired label technique for testing mouse myeloma proteins. In this method, aliquots of purified rabbit anti-mouse myeloma protein labelled with iodine-125 and normal rabbit serum labelled with iodine-131 were added to cell lines and the binding of each was enumerated and compared.

Since these early reports, RIA in tumour immunology has been adapted to include all the liquid- and solid-phase assays described earlier, not only for detecting antibody to tumours, but also tumour-specific antigens and tumour viruses.

The detection of tumour antigen and viruses is beyond the scope of this book, but it is worth noting that such techniques have proved useful as indicators of the presence of tumour tissue (as a serological screening test), and also for the preparation of specific antibody. Antibodies prepared in this way can be used in competitive binding assays to measure the patients antibody to the tumour (i.e. diagnostically), or after attachment of cytotoxic substances to the antibodies they may be used in treatment. Similarly, attempts have been made with radiolabelled tumour-specific antibody to locate the site of a tumour by injection of the material followed by scanning.

While RIA techniques for tumour antibody do not vary substantially from those already described, it should be pointed out that RIA has certain advantages over other methods. For example, cytotoxicity tests frequently used in tumour work are often of limited value because some antibodies do not have cytotoxic characteristics. For the RIA this is not a disadvantage, and the assay does not require complement, which is always a constant source of standardization difficulties. RIA is easily adaptable to the detection of antibody by cells grown in tissue culture, adherent cells, cells in suspension or antibody to tissues which have been taken from the tumour-bearing host. In addition, the Fc portion of the antiglobulin molecule may be removed to prevent the interference caused by binding of this part of the molecule to cellular receptors. A further advantage is that one antiglobulin reagent may be used in the detection of antibody in an indirect assay, thus allowing direct comparison with the need for only one standardization procedure. Finally, live cells may be used as antigens without fear of interference by cellular enzymes as is the case with enzyme-linked immunosorbent assays (ELISA). This is a definite advantage because chemical or physical treatment of cells to kill them often results in the destruction or modification of antigens.

130

Antibody to experimentally used antigens

The application of RIA for the detection of antibody to antigens used experimentally depends largely on the nature of the antigen. However, RIA techniques can be designed for use with almost any antigen and much more can be learned by the use of RIA than by the use of conventional tests. Although conventional tests are still widely used in experimental work, it is strongly suggested that a primary binding assay should be used if possible. Some reference to the use of RIA of antibody in clinical research has already been made (see Chapter 7).

One of the most frequently used antigens in experimental immunology is the sheep erythrocyte. Antibody production to this antigen has been shown to depend on thymus-derived lymphocytes, which makes it a valuable agent for immunological research. It is readily available (commercially) and may be stored for an extended period if treated with formalin or glutaraldehyde. Antibody to sheep erythrocytes can be detected by an agglutination test, and as such can be roughly quantitated by a double dilution test of sera. The contribution of IgM and non-agglutinating IgG (or other immunoglobulin classes) may be estimated by using a reducing agent such as 2-mercaptoethanol, which removes any agglutination activity due to IgM. The contribution of IgG antibody can be established by a Coombs-type indirect agglutination test. Both of these methods, however, are inaccurate and at best provide only an approximate measure of the levels of antibody. The main advantages of the agglutination test are its technical ease and the fact that it may be performed in any laboratory without expensive equipment.

If RIA was used in the detection of antibody to this particulate antigen, a number of factors would have to be considered. The foremost of these is the type of information required, including:

(a) Whether a comparison of antibody levels or quantitation is necessary. If a comparison is wanted, counts per minute of antiglobulin bound would suffice. If, however, quantitation of antibody is required, a second procedure to relate the bound radiolabelled antiglobulin and antibody is needed. This may be achieved in several ways, the two most popular being acid elution of bound antibody from the antigen followed by measurement of the amount of eluted antibody, or by the use of a purified immunoglobulin bound to a solid matrix (see Chapter 5)

(b) Whether the contribution of each of the immunoglobulin classes to the antibody response is required instead of a global estimate. For a global antibody measurement, an antiglobulin reagent with antibody activity to all the immunoglobulin classes is required. In this instance care must be taken to ascertain that antibody to all the classes is present in excess amounts or error will result. For example, early in the antibody response large amounts of IgM antibody are produced. Unless the antiglobulin reagent has a substantial reactivity with IgM or a large amount of conjugate is used, erroneously low results may be obtained because insufficient anti-IgM antibody is present. To overcome this difficulty, it is recommended that two or three dilutions of test serum, apart by a factor of ten, are used. A linear relationship between dilution and counts per minute should be obtained. For assessing the contribution of antibody of each immunoglobulin class to the response, heavy-chain specific antisera are required. These may either be radiolabelled directly or an anti-species globulin conjugated to an isotope may be used for an indirect or amplified technique. The advantage of the former is that it is technically simpler, but it requires several radiolabelled antisera. The advantages of the indirect method are that it requires only one radiolabelled reagent and the sensitivity is increased. It is again recommended that dilutions of test sera be used in either assay to ascertain antigen and antiglobulin excess.

Other considerations

Most of these have been covered in other chapters and include the need for replicate tests and the inclusion of a standard positive, a low-titred serum and several negative sera. Also, sources of error, apart from those due to lack of excess of antigen and antiglobulin, must be considered. Such errors include the presence of rheumatoid factor in the sera and immunoglobulin attached non-specifically to the erythrocyte antigen.

Many researchers, of course, utilize soluble antigens, not particulate ones as in the above. In these cases the soluble antigens may be used in RIA procedures either by rendering them insoluble and using an assay as outlined above or by performing a liquid-type assay as described earlier in the chapter.

Although it is realized that the apparent technical difficulties of RIA procedures may appear problematical, it should be borne in mind that the data obtained using these sensitive techniques are more accurate, more reproducible and provide more detail than can be gained by conventional serological tests.

ANTIBODY TO DRUGS

It has been known for many years that one of the best ways of assaying drugs is to use a competitive radioimmunoassay. Examples of drugs which are measured in this way include gentamicin and digoxin, and in all instances where such a method is used it is necessary first to obtain a specific antibody. Experience has shown that antibodies are not easily produced against small molecules such as these, but if the drug is attached to carrier protein, antibody production is possible. Similarly, when drugs are administered they may attach to 'carriers' in the body and therefore provide a stimulus for antibody production. This is an unexplored area but there are well known examples where an antibody response to a bound drug causes tissue damage and therefore disease. One such example is the now notorious hypnotic Sedormid, which attaches to platelets and leads to an immune destruction of these cells, with subsequent purpura. Another example is of the attachment of antibiotics, notably penicillins, to polymorphonuclear leucocytes, with subsequent destruction of these cells (Weitzman *et al.*, 1978).

However, the use of assays, and particularly radioimmunoassays, to measure antibody produced to drugs has not received much attention. That the method can be extremely useful is shown by the example below, which is drawn from our own experience (McKenzie *et al.*, 1976). In this study we investigated the nature of rashes which occur following the administration of ampicillin to patients with infectious mononucleosis. It was considered that this rash must have an immunological (i.e. hypersensitivity) basis, and an attempt was made to demonstrate antibody to this drug. The assay used was a direct antibody assay in which the drug was coupled to cyanogen bromide-activated Sephadex® (see Chapter 2), and reacted with the patient's serum and then with radiolabelled anti-human IgG or anti-human IgM. The study indicated that although antibody to ampicillin could be demonstrated in many 'normals', the levels of IgM and IgG antibody to the drug were many times higher in patients with infectious mononucleosis and this was unrelated to the administration of the drug. In other words, the disease itself had stimulated the antibody production, and any subsequent administration of the drug had secondarily produced the hypersensitivity. A further interesting and useful application of this particular assay was that it showed the value of RIA antibody in testing the specificity of a reaction. This aspect, important to the researcher, is often difficult to examine. In the above instance of ampicillin reactivity, it was possible to show that the specificity was for this drug alone, and not for other members of the penicillin family, or for cephalosporins which are closely related. This differentiation was achieved by adding equivalent amounts of different drugs (e.g. cloxacillin, penicillin, carbenicillin) to the standard assay of antibody and observing the reduction in activity due to competition. The greatest competition was with ampicillin and most of the other drugs produced little competitive activity.

The results showed that an assay *for ampicillin* could be achieved in this way, although it was not the purpose of the study to do that, just as it is not the purpose of this book to consider assays of 'antigens'.

Nevertheless, the point must be made that the measurement of antibody to drugs may be an increasingly important part of modern therapeutic management, and ignorance of this area may be leading to a failure to recognize some important consequences of therapy.

REFERENCES

Arendt, J., Paunier, L., and Sizonenko, P. C. (1975). Melatonin radioimmunoassay. *J. Clin. Endocrinol. Metab.*, **40**, 347–350.

Beeken, W. L., and Roessner, K. D. (1975). Radioimmunoassay of human jejunal IgA secretion. *Proc. Soc. Exp. Biol. Med.*, **148**, 739–742.

Bennett, R. M., and Mohla, C. (1976). A solid-phase radioimmunoassay for the measurement of lactoferrin in human plasma: variations with age, sex and disease. *J. Lab. Clin. Med.*, **88**, 156–166.

Butler, V. P., Jr. (1975). Drug immunoassays. *J. Immunol. Methods*, **7**, 1–24.

133

Catt, K., Niall, H. D., and Tregear, G. W. (1966). Solid-phase radioimmunoassay of human growth hormone. *Biochem. J.*, **100**, 31 and 33c.

Claus, D. R., Osmond, A. P., and Gewurz, H. (1976). Radioimmunoassay of human C-reactive protein and levels in normal sera. *J. Lab. Clin. Med.*, **87**, 120–128.

Duimel, W. J., and Brummelhuis, H. G. (1975). A new solid-phase radioimmunoassay (CLB-RIA) for the detection of hepatitis-B antigen and antibody. *Vox. Sang.*, **29**, 1–14.

Forrester, P. I., Hancock, R. L., Hay, D. M., Lai, P. C. W., and Lorscheider, F. L. (1975). A rapid method for the purification and radioimmunoassay of human alpha-fetoprotein. *Clin. Chim. Acta*, **64**, 317–323.

Fránek, M., and Hruska, K. J. (1976). Separation of free and protein-bound ligands in the radioimmunoassay by gel filtration–centrifugation. *J. Chromatogr.*, **119**, 167–172.

Harder, F. H., and McKhann, C. F. (1968). Demonstration of cellular antigens on sarcoma cells by an indirect [125]-I-labelled antibody technique. *J. Nat. Cancer Inst.*, **40**, 231–245.

Herrmann, J. E., and Collins, M. F. (1976). Quantitation of immunoglobulin adsorption to plastics. *J. Immunol. Methods*, **10**, 363–366.

Hutchinson, H. D., and Ziegler, D. W. (1972). Simplified radioimmunoassay for diagnostic serology. *Appl. Microbiol.*, **24**, 742–749.

Kalimo, K. O., Ziola, B. R., Viljanen, M. K. Granfors, K., and Toivanen, P. (1977). Solid-phase radioimmunoassay of herpes simplex virus of IgG and IgM antibodies. *J. Immunol. Methods*, **14**, 183–195.

Kida, S., and Muller-Eberhard, U. (1975). A radioimmunoassay employing polyethylene glycol (PEG) for measuring dilute concentrations of rat hemopexin, albumin and haptoglobulin. *Immunochemistry*, **12**, 97–99.

Kleinberg, D. L. (1975). Human alpha-lactalbumin: measurement in serum and in breast cancer organ cultures by radioimmunoassay. *Science*, **190**, 276–278.

Ling, C. M., and Overby, L. R. (1972). Prevalence of hepatitis B virus antigen as revealed by direct radioimmune assay with [125]-I-antibody. *J. Immunol.*, **109**, 834–841.

Luxton, A. W., Walker, W. J. Gauldie, J., Ali, M. A. M., and Pelletier, C. (1977). A radioimmunoassay for serum ferritin. *Clin. Chem.*, **23**, 683–689.

McKenzie, H., Parratt, D., and White, R. G. (1976). IgM and IgG antibody levels to ampicillin in patients with infectious mononucleosis. *Clin. Exp. Immunol.*, **26**, 214–221.

Nerenberg, S. T., and Prasad, R. (1975). Radioimmunoassays for Ig classes G, A, M, D and E in spinal fluids normal values of different age groups. *J. Lab. Clin. Med.*, **86**, 887–898.

Plesner, T., Nörgaard-Pedersen, B., and Boenisch, T. (1975). Radioimmunoassay of beta-2-microglobulin. *Scand. J. Clin. Lab. Invest.*, **35**, 729–735.

Reif, A. E. (1971). A quantitative assay for cell bound antibody using a radiolabelled Coombs-type antiserum to a gamma G myeloma protein. *J. Immunol.*, **106**, 573–575.

Saito, H., Ratnoff, O. D., and Pensky, J. (1976). Radioimmunoassay of human Hagemen factor (Factor XII). *J. Lab. Clin. Med.*, **88**, 506–514.

Schieble, J. H., and Cottam, D. (1977). Solid-phase radioimmunoassay as a method for evaluating antigenic differences in type A influenza viruses. *Infect. Immunol.*, **15**, 66–71.

Skelley, D. S., Brown, L. P., and Besch, P. K. (1973). Radioimmunoassay. *Clin. Chem.*, **19**, 146–186.

Tanigaki, N. Yagi, Y., Moore, G. E., and Pressman, D. (1966). Immunoglobulin production in human leukemia cell lines. *J. Immunol.*, **97**, 634–646.

Taniguchi, N., Tanaka, M., Kobayashi, K., Matsuda, I., Ohno, H., Sato, T., and Takakuwa, E. (1976). A solid-phase radioimmunoassay for human beta-2-microglobulin. *Clin. Chim. Acta*, **69**, 471–477.

Taubman, S. B., Cogen, R. B., and Lepow, I. H. (1974). Granule enzymes from human leukocytes: their effect on HeLa cells. *Proc. Soc. Exp. Biol. Med.*, **145**, 952–957.

Ting, C. C., and Herberman, R. B. (1971). Inverse relationship of polyoma tumour specific cell surface antigen to H-2 histocompatibility antigens. *Nature New Biol.*, **232**, 118–120.

134

Vincent, C., and Revillar, J. P. (1976). Comparison of radioimmunoassay and lymphocytotoxicity inhibition techniques for the determination of beta-2-microglobulin. *J. Immunol. Methods*, **10**, 253–259.

Weitzman, S. A., Stossel, T. P., and Desmond, M. (1978). Drug-induced immunological neutropenia. *Lancet*, **1**, 1068.

Wide, L. (1969). Radioimmunoassays employing immunosorbents. *Acta Endocrinol. (Copenhagen)*, **142** (Suppl.) 207–221.

Chapter 9

Radioimmunoassay of antibody in veterinary medicine

INTRODUCTION

Veterinary diagnostics and medical research involving experimental animals are areas where RIA has apparently found only limited application in the past. One of the problems is that the use of several test species requires a large variety of antisera and, because radiolabelled antisera cannot be stored for long periods, the use of RIA is less feasible. Further, diagnostic use of RIA for a large number of samples within a single species, which is typical in veterinary work, often requires automation which, although possible, is difficult at present with many of the RIAs described in this book. Another area of concern in the use of RIA in veterinary medicine is expense. Thus, it is a relatively expensive procedure compared with an agglutination test, even though it is more efficient. The extra cost is due mainly to the reagents and equipment required, whereas the reagents for mass serology require additional and continuous standardization, which can be difficult for the laboratory (see Chapter 5 on standardization). Further, in some animals such as cattle, where RIA may be of use, natural antibody may interfere with the assay. These problems will be discussed below in more detail.

Despite these difficulties, RIA has found and will continue to find uses in veterinary medicine. Probably owing to its economic importance, the serology of cattle has been the area most exploited by RIA, closely followed by that of chickens.

USE OF RIA IN CATTLE SEROLOGY

Literature references for RIA of antibodies to a wide variety of aetiological agents are available, but before discussing the methods we should introduce a caution with regard to bovine serum proteins.

Natural antibodies are frequently present in cattle to a large number of antigens, a simple example being the well known bovine antibody to sheep

135

136

Table 9.1. Natural antibody to *Brucella abortus*
in several species

Animal	Agglutination titre range*
Guinea-pig	1:4
Rabbit	1:4
Sheep	1:16–1:65
Goat	1:4–1:16
Cow	1:4–1:2048
Horse	1:16–1:64
Pig	1:16–1:64
Human	1:4–1:64

*These are titres obtained from sera in the absence of
any evidence of brucellosis.

erythrocytes. Such an antibody is not likely to lead to many diagnostic difficulties but, where the natural antibody reacts with the antigens of a microorganism, problems arise.

Table 9.1 lists some of the species which have natural antibody to *B. abortus*. Different cattle sera have variable titres (determined by agglutination) and there are sera which contain a very high titre to this bacterium in the absence of any other evidence of brucellosis. Such a high titre would normally be diagnostically significant. The natural antibody has been found to be mainly IgM in type but often contains minute amounts of IgG. To avoid false-positive serological reactions caused by these natural antibodies, it would be possible and preferable to use an assay which measures only IgG (IgG_1 and IgG_2 subclasses) antibody. Primary binding assays should be useful for this purpose as the specificity of the antibody classes measured can be predetermined by the specificity of the conjugate used. The problem, however, is that detection of IgM antibody early in *B. abortus* infection is *useful* and by excluding the measurement of IgM in serological assays (Chapters 1 and 7), animals with early infection may be missed. In contrast, inclusion of IgM measurement would lead to a number of false-positive results.

This dilemma remains at present but it should be pointed out that with primary binding assays such as RIA or ELISA the choice of measurement of IgM separately from IgG exists. This is not the case using secondary antibody assays such as the complement fixation test, which measures IgM and IgG_1, but excludes IgG_2 because of its inability to bind guinea-pig complement. Similarly, agglutination tests at neutral pH tend to measure IgM and IgG_2 antibody to the exclusion of IgG_1, whereas agglutination tests at an acidic pH measure IgG but exclude IgM indiscriminately. Another difficulty with some secondary antibody assays is the occurrence of a prozone, a phenomenon not seen with RIA (in antigen excess) but observed in ELISA (with limited antigen) in the presence of very high IgM levels.

Indeed, the major difficulty in most ELISA assays is that of achieving antigen excess. Often this is either not realized, or not reported by the investigator, despite the fact that a failure in this respect means that the assay will perform no better than conventional 'secondary' binding tests.

The preparation of heavy-chain specific antisera for bovine immunoglobulins has been greatly facilitated by the finding that guinea pigs immunized with complete immunoglobulin molecules (from bovines) do not produce antibody to the light chains. Thus anti-bovine IgM and IgA can be prepared easily with little or no absorption needed to attain monospecificity. Preparation of anti-bovine IgG_1 or IgG_2 is more complicated because the heavy chains of these immunoglobulins cross-react, and normally reciprocal absorption is necessary. Bovine IgG_2 can be simply prepared by anion-exchange chromatography and therefore absorption of anti-IgG_1 is straightforward (Duncan et al., 1972). However, IgG_1 is not easy to purify, making absorption of anti-IgG_2 antiserum difficult. In our experience, this difficulty can be overcome by intravenous injection of whole goat serum into the guinea pigs immediately prior to immunization with bovine IgG_2. About 60% of the annals will then produce monospecific anti-IgG_2 antibody. This does not seem to be the case for IgG_1 antibody production.

An alternative method for obtaining anti-IgG_2 would be to prepare IgG_2 as noted above and to purify the antiserum by affinity chromatography (Chapter 3). The amount of antiserum required will in many cases determine which method is the most practical.

Chapter 3 did not consider the production of antiserum in guinea-pigs, and the preparation of antisera to bovine globulins in these animals is considered briefly here. Adult albino SPF guinea-pigs should be immunized by injecting 0.1 ml of antigen emulsified in Freund's complete adjuvant into the four footpads. The 0.4 ml of immunizing material should contain 0.1–1.0 mg of antigen. The animals are injected again 2 weeks later with the same antigen dose (0.1–1.0 mg total) in complete Freund's adjuvant intramuscularly (into the gluteus maximus). Bleeding, usually by cardiac puncture, should be carried out 1 week after the second injection. In this way good anti-heavy chain specific antisera to bovine immunoglobulins can be prepared in 3 weeks. Alternatively, the rabbit is useful for the preparation of anti-bovine globulin antiserum (Coomb's reagent). In this case, 5 weeks should separate the primary and secondary injections (see Chapter 3). Sheep have not been found to be satisfactory for anti-bovine antiserum preparation, whereas goats are useful because of the large serum volume obtained. Goats, however, generally produce a weaker antiserum than do guinea-pigs and absorption is necessary. It is recognized that guinea-pigs are expensive to purchase but the extra expense is usually compensated for by the short duration of the immunization procedure and the decreased handling of the antisera to make them heavy-chain specific.

Bacterial serology in cattle

Brucellosis and mycobacterial infections are probably the most important bacterial diseases of cattle, and RIA procedures for antibody have been used which are different from the direct assay in human serology discussed in Chapter 7. Chappel *et al.* (1976, 1978) devised an RIA procedure which used whole *B. abortus* cells as the antigen and ^{125}I-labelled bovine anti-Brucella IgG$_1$ to compete with binding by antibody in serum. Bovine anti-Brucella IgG$_2$ was found to compete as well as IgG$_1$ for binding, but IgM did not. The authors found a good correlation between the RIA and the complement fixation test. A particular advantage of the RIA was its ability to distinguish between antibody responses of infected and vaccinated cattle, a long-standing and troublesome aspect of brucellosis serology. This solid-phase direct competition RIA should be of considerable value in diagnostic serology and should have an assured future. The one limitation is the need for a purified bovine anti-Brucella IgG. Modern methods of affinity chromatography should, however, overcome this difficulty, even if they are laborious.

A second type of RIA for bovine brucellosis has been described by Levieux (1978). This carefully conducted study made use of whole-cell antigen which was bound to glass tubes by drying and fixation with alcohol. With this assay there was no need for centrifugation, thus removing a time-consuming and tedious aspect of the standard solid-phase direct RIA. In our hands, however, some difficulties have been encountered through loss of bound antigen in the washing procedures. These technical difficulties can probably be overcome and the method promises to become valuable in diagnosis.

Surprisingly, no literature is available on the use of soluble *B. abortus* antigen attached to a cellulose or other solid phase in RIA of bovine serology, but it should be possible. Wilson *et al.* (1977) gave a general discussion of antigen attachment to solid-phase materials (see also Chapter 2).

The use of whole-cell antigen may not be desirable owing to cross-reaction with antibody to *Yersinia enterocolitica* serotype 0 : 99. The specificity of assays could be increased by eliminating such cross-reacting antigenic determinants, and this might be achieved by using a purified and separated antigen. Often, though, the soluble antigens which promise increased specificity do not lend themselves to radiolabelling or attachment to a solid matrix. Thus, a solid-phase RIA used by Wilson *et al.* (1977) for antigen detection could perhaps be modified for serological procedures. In addition to these assays, the direct solid-phase RIA method similar to that described in Chapter 7 has been used by Rurangirwa (1979) and by Nielsen *et al.* (1978) for bovine *B. abortus* serology.

RIA procedures similar to the Farr technique (see Chapter 4) have been described for mycobacterial antigens. Minden and Farr (1969) obtained inconclusive results with *Mycobacterium tuberculosis* antigen. On the other hand, Worsaae (1978), using ^{125}I-labelled *M. paratuberculosis* PPD as an antigen, found this type of assay very useful.

If direct assay of antibody to mycobacterial antigens is to be used, Freund's complete adjuvant should not be used for antiserum (i.e. antiglobulin) production as this contains *M. tuberculosis*, and antibody formed against this component interferes in the assay.

Because the number of samples to be handled may be large, and may require large amounts of isotope, RIA may not be the best choice in bovine serology, although it should be noted that production of a good antiglobulin by affinity chromatography (Chapter 3) allows less radioisotope to be used without altering the sensitivity and specificity of the assays.

Viral serology in cattle

RIA has been applied successfully to the detection of both antigen and antibody to bovine leukosis virus (BLV). A major structural component of BLV-24 can be purified, radiolabelled and used in the detection of antibody. This assay was shown to be specific for BLV as antisera to other mamalian RNA tumour viruses did not cross-react. Similarly, using a specific antiserum and radiolabelled p24 antigen, the presence of antigen p24 in tissue culture can be detected. These RIA procedures were shown to be more sensitive than indirect fluorescence and gel diffusion tests (Devare et al., 1976; McDonald and Ferrer, 1976). A solid-phase RIA procedure has also been developed for detection of antibody to bovine rotavirus (neonatal calf diarrhoea) by Babiuk et al. (1977).

Parasitic and other antigens

An RIA procedure has been developed for the detection of antibody to *Fasciola gigantica* in cattle sera (Bitakaramire et al., 1971).

In a different area, RIA has been used to study catabolic rates of immunoglobulins and complement components of cattle (Nielsen et al., 1978) and for the measurement of total reaginic antibody of cattle (Nielsen, 1977; Wilkie et al., 1978).

OTHER VETERINARY APPLICATIONS

Although it is evident that the application of RIA to veterinary serology is in its infancy, several RIA procedures, not varying greatly from those already described, have been devised. For completion but to avoid repetition, a referenced list of applications is provided in Table 9.2.

FUTURE TRENDS IN VETERINARY SEROLOGY

There has been a plethora of reports dealing with hormone and drug measurements by RIA in veterinary medicine, but RIA has not found widespread use in the detection of antibody. In our view, there are a number of reasons for this, the principal one of which is the diversity of species and therefore the diversity of antiserum conjugates involved. This problem is particularly troublesome when antibody of different immunoglobulin types is to be measured. On the other hand, the effort is worthwhile because veterinary medicine is vitally important globally and, in addition, animal experiments are frequently used by the researcher of human problems, particularly in the elucidation of basic

140

Table 9.2. Applications of RIA procedures in veterinary serology

Antigen	Species	Literature reference
Bacterial:		
Salmonella sp.	Chicken	White and Nielsen (1975)
Viral:		
Avian leukosis virus	Chicken	Chen and Hanafusa (1974); Sandelin *et al.* (1974)
Avian oncornavirus	Chicken	Stephenson *et al.* (1973); Bosch *et al.* (1978); Collins *et al.* (1978); Higuchi and August (1977)
Newcastle disease virus	Chicken	Spira *et al.* (1976a, b); Cleland *et al.* (1975)
Marek's disease virus	Chicken	
African swine fever	Swine	Crowther *et al.* (1977)
C type virus	Cat/mouse	Scolnick *et al.* (1972)
	Mink	Barbacid *et al.* (1978)
Western equine encephalomyelitis	Rabbit	Levitt *et al.* (1976)
Rabies virus	Rabbit, man	Wiktor *et al.* (1972); Lee (1976); Bruns *et al.* (1977); Lee *et al.* (1977)
Foot-and-mouth disease	(Serotyping)	Crowther (1977)
Parasitic and other antigens:		
Toxoplasmosis	Man	Gehle *et al.* (1976)
Alpha-fetoprotein	Sheep	Lai *et al.* (1978)
Secretory alloantigens	Dog	Oriol *et al.* (1975)

immunology. It is therefore of importance that the most accurate and sensitive methodology be available for serological studies and diagnosis. Fortunately, a number of approaches are available for simplifying RIA procedures which are to be used for different species, and these are listed below.

Use of cross-reacting antiglobulins

A number of different species cross-react extensively in the specificity of immunoglobulins. For example, anti-bovine immunoglobulin reagents can be used to detect antibody of the goat and a variety of other ruminants. Similarly, anti-chicken reagents are of value with sera from other avian species. Therefore, if no antisera are available for one species a reasonable alternative would be to attempt to use antisera prepared for immunoglobulins of a related species. Although this is a derogation of scientific principle, it may be useful as a practical measure, but the sensitivity and accuracy of the assay are unlikely to be as high as they would be with the appropriate reagents.

Use of double antiglobulin methods

An anti-anti-immunoglobulin reagent can be used to eliminate the requirement of radiolabelling individual anti-heavy-chain antisera and also for increasing the usefulness of the reagents between species. For example, guinea-pig anti-bovine IgM, IgA, IgG$_1$ and IgG$_2$ antisera can be detected with a radiolabelled rabbit anti-guinea pig globulin and the same anti-guinea-pig reagent can be used to detect guinea-pig anti-porcine immunoglobulin antisera. Thus, one radiolabelled preparation may be used for at least eight different tests. In addition, this indirect–indirect type of assay increases the sensitivity of the RIA by amplifying the number of radiolabelled molecules attached to the primary antigen–antibody–antiglobulin complex (see Chapter 5).

Use of staphylococcal protein A

Staphylococcus aureus protein A interacts with the Fc portion of immunoglobulins from many species. (Goudswaard *et al.*, 1978). Therefore, radiolabelled protein A may be used in place of antiglobulins as the detection reagent in RIA. Several methods making use of this property of protein A are available (Langone *et al.*, 1977; Brunda *et al.*, 1977; Moran *et al.*, 1978) and may be of interest in RIA applications in veterinary medicine.

REFERENCES

Babiuk, L. A., Acres, S. D., and Rouse, B. T. (1977). Solid-phase radioimmunoassay for detecting bovine (neonatal calf diarrhoea) rotavirus antibody. *J. Clin. Microbiol.*, **6**, 10–15.

Barbacid, M., Trowick, S. R., and Aaronson, S. A. (1978). Isolation and characterisation of an endogenous type C RNA virus of mink (MvlLu) cells. *J. Virol.*, **25**, 129–137.

Bitakaramire, P. K., Movesesijam, M., and Castelino, J. B. (1971). Radioimmunoassay for *Fasciola gigantica* infection in cattle. *Bull. Epizoot. Dis. Afr.*, **19**, 353–356.

Bosch, V., Kurth, R., and Smart, J. E. (1978). The detection of glycoproteins immunologically related to RSV gp85 in uninfected avian cells and in sera from uninfected birds. *Virology*, **86**, 226–240.

Brunda, M. J., Minden, P., Sharpton, T. R., McClatchy, J. K., and Farr, R. S. (1977). Precipitation of radiolabelled antigen–antibody complexes with protein-A containing *Staphylococcus aureus*. *J. Immunol.*, **119**, 193–198.

Brunner, H., Schaeg, W., Bruck, U., Schummer, U., Sziegoleit, D., and Schiefer, H. G. Detection of IgG, IgM and IgA antibodies to *Mycoplasma pneumoniae* by an indirect staphylococcal radioimmunoassay. *Med. Microbiol. Immunol.*, **165**, 29–41. (1978).

Bruns, M., Dietzschold, B., Schneider, L. G., and Cox, J. H. (1977). Comparison of the ribonucleoproteins of different rabies virus serotypes by radioimmunoassay. *J. Immunol. Methods*, **18**, 337–346.

Chappel, R. J., Williamson, P., McNaught, D. J., Dalling, M. J., and Allan, G. S. (1976). Radioimmunoassay for antibodies against *Brucella abortus*: a new serological test for bovine brucellosis. *J. Hyg.*, **77**, 369–376.

Chappel, R. J., McNaught, D. J., Bourke, J. A., and Allan G. S. (1978). The diagnostic efficiency of some serological tests for bovine brucellosis. *J. Hyg.*, **80**, 373–384.

Chen, J. H., and Hanafusa, H. (1974). Detection of a protein of avian leukoviruses in uninfected chick cells by radioimmuno-assay. *J. Virol.*, **13**, 340–346.

Cleland, G. B., Perey, D. Y. E., and Dent, P. B. (1975). Micro-radioimmunoassay for antibodies to Newcastle disease virus in the chicken. *J. Immunol.*, **114**, 422–425.

Collins, J. J., Montelaro, R. C., Denny, T. B., Ishizaka, R., Langlois, A. J., and Golognesi, D. P. (1978). Normal chicken cells express a surface antigen which cross-reacts with determinants of the major envelope glycoprotein of avian myeloblastosis virus. *Virology*, **86**, 205–216.

Crowther, J. R. (1977). Examination of differences between foot-and-mouth disease virus strains using a radioimmunoassay technique, in *Proc. Int. Symp. Foot-and-Mouth Dis. II*, (Eds. C. Mackowiak and R. H. Reganny, Karger, Basle, pp. 185–193.

Devare, S. G., Stephenson, J. R., Sarma, P. S., Aaronson, S. A., and Chander, S. (1976). Bovine lymphosarcoma: development of a radioimmunologic technique for detection of the etiologic agent. *Science*, **194**, 1428–1430.

Duncan, J. R., Wilkie, B. N., Hiestand, F., and Winter, A. J. (1972). Serum and secretory immunoglobulins of cattle: characterisation and quantitation. *J. Immunol.*, **108**, 965–976.

Gehle, W. D., Smith, K. O., and Fuccillo, D. A. (1976). Radioimmunoassay for toxoplasmosis. *Infect. Immun.*, **14**, 1252–1255.

Goudswaard, J., Van der Douk, J. A., Noordzij, A., van Dam, R. H., and Vaerman, J. P. (1978). Protein A reactivity of various mammalian immunoglobulins. *Scand. J. Immunol.*, **8**, 21–28.

Higuchi, T., and August, J. T. (1977). Characterisation of tumor virus proteins. I. Radioimmunoassay of the p27 protein of avian viruses. *Rev. Bras. Pesqui. Med.*, **10**, 1–14.

Lai, P. C. W., Hay, D. M., and Lorscheider, F. L. (1978). Radioimmunoassay of ovine alpha-fetoprotein. *J. Immunol. Methods*, **20**, 1–10.

Langone, J. J., Boyle, M. D. P., and Borsos, T. (1977). ^{125}I protein A: application to the quantitative determination of fluid phase and cell-bound IgG. *J. Immunol.*, **18**, 281–293.

Langone, J. J. (1978). (^{125}I) protein A: a tracer for general use in immunoassay. *J. Immunol. Methods*, **24**, 269–285.

Lee, T.-K. (1976). Detection of rabies antigen and antibody by direct and indirect radioimmunoassay. *Diss. Abstr. Int. B.*, **36**, 4865.

Lee, T.-K., Hutchinson, H. D., and Ziegler, D. W. (1977). Comparison of rabies humoral antibody titers in rabbits and humans by indirect radioimmunoassay, rapid-fluorescent-focus inhibition technique and indirect fluorescent antibody assay. *J. Clin. Microbiol.*, **5**, 320–325.

Levieux, D. (1978). A solid-phase radioimmunoassay for the determination of bacterial specific antibodies within different immunoglobulin classes: application to bovine *Brucella aborus* antibodies. *Ann. Rech. Vet.*, **9**, 523–530.

Levitt, N. H., Miller, H. V., and Eddy, G. A. (1976). Solid-phase radioimmunoassay for rapid detection and identification of western equine encephalomyelitis virus. *J. Clin. Microbiol.*, **4**, 382–383.

McDonald, H. C., and Ferrer, J. F. (1976). Detection, quantitation and characterisation of the major internal virion antigen of the bovine leukaemia virus by radioimmunoassay. *J. Nat. Cancer Inst.*, **57**, 875–882.

Minden, P., and Farr, R. S. (1969). Binding between components of the tubercle bacillus and humoral antibodies. *J. Exp. Med.*, **130**, 931–954.

Moran, D. M., Dupe, B. E., and Gauntlett, S. (1978). A microimmunoassay method for measuring IgG antibodies using Staphylococcal protein A. *J. Immunol. Methods*, **24**, 183–191.

Nielsen, K. H. (1977). Bovine reaginic antibody. III. Cross-reaction of anti-human IgE and antibovine reaginic immuno-globulin antisera with sera from several species of mammals. *Can. J. Comp. Med.*, **41**, 345–348.

Nielsen, K. H., Sheppard, J., Holmes, W., and Tizard, I. (1978). Experimental bovine trypanosomiasis. Changes in the catabolism of serum immunoglobulins and complement components in infected cattle. *Immunology*, **35**, 811–816.

Nielsen, K. H., Duncan, J. R., and Stemshorn, B. (1980). Relationship of humoral factors (antibody and complement) in immune responsiveness, resistance and diagnostic serology, in *Proc. Int. Symp. Ruminant Immunol.* (Ed. J. E. Butler), Plenum Press, New York.

Oriol, R., Strecker, G., Rousset, M., Chevalier, G., Dalix, A. M., Dussaulx, D. E., and Zweibaum, A. (1975). Determination of the structure of the immunodominant groups of canine secretory allo-antigens (CSA) by radioimmunoassay. *Transplant Proc.*, **7**, 523–528.

Rurangirwa, F. (1979). Immunosuppression during *Trypanosoma coagolense* and *Trypanosoma vivax* infections in Zebu cattle (*Bos. indicus*). PhD Thesis, University of Guelph, Guelph, Ont., Canada.

Sandelin, K., Estola, T., Ristimaki, S., Ruoslahti, E., and Valeri, A. (1974). Radio-immunoassay of the group-specific antigen in detection of avian leukosis virus infection. *J. Gen. Virol.*, **25**, 415–420.

Scolnick, E. M., Parks, W. P., and Livingston, D. M. (1972). Radioimmunoassay of mammalian type C viral proteins. I. Species specific reactions of murine and feline viruses. *J. Immunol.*, **109**, 570–577.

Soergel, M. F., Schaffer, F. L., Sawyer, J. C., and Prato, C. M. (1978). Assay of antibodies to caliciviruses by radioimmune precipitation using staphylococcal protein A as IgG adsorbent. *Arch. Virol.*, **57**, 271–282.

Spira, G., Silvian, I., and Zakay-Roues, Z. (1976a). Detection of Newcastle disease virus antigen and antibodies by the aid of radioimmunoassay. *Israel J. Med. Sci.*, **12**, 713–714.

Spira, G., Silvian, I., and Zakay-Roues, Z. (1976b). Radioimmunoassay for detection of antigen and antibodies to Newcastle disease virus. *J. Immunol.*, **116**, 1089–1092.

Stephenson, J. R., Wilsnack, R. E., and Aaronson, S. A. (1973). Radioimmunoassay for avian C-type virus group-specific antigen: detection in normal and virus-transformed cells. *J. Virol.*, **11**, 893–899.

White, R. G., and Nielsen, K. H. (1975). Interactions between the immunological responses of a thymus-dependent antigen (*Salmonella adelaide* C. antigen) with the thymus-dependent antigen (sheep erythrocytes) in the adult bird. *Immunology*, **28**, 959–972.

Wiktor, T. J., Koprowski, H., and Dixon, F. (1972). Radioimmunoassay procedure in rabies binding antibodies. *J. Immunol.*, **109**, 464–479.

Wilkie, B. N., Nielsen, K. H., and Little, J. (1978). Experimental hypersensitivity pneumonitis: serum immunoglobulins G_1, G_2, M, A and E in *Micropolyspora faeni* sensitised and de-sensitised calves. *Int. Arch. Allergy Appl. Immunol.*, **56**, 79–86.

Wilson, D. V., Thornley, M. J., and Coombs, R. R. A. (1977). A solid-phase assay with radioactivity-labelled antibody for the detection of *Brucella abortus*. *J. Med. Microbiol.*, **10**, 281–292.

Worsaae, H. (1978). Radioimmunoassay for antibodies against *Mycobacterium paratuberculosis* using ^{125}I-labelled PPD. *Acta Vet. Scand.*, **19**, 153–155.

Appendix

BUFFERS

1. 0.1 M phosphate buffer (pH 7.2)

Add 28 ml of 0.2 M monobasic sodium phosphate ($NaH_2 PO_4$, 27.8 g/l) to 72 ml of 0.2 M dibasic sodium phosphate ($Na_2 HPO_4$. $7H_2O$, 53.65 g/l, or $Na_2 HPO_4$. $10H_2O$, 71.7 g/l). Dilute the mixture with 100 ml of distilled water to a final volume of 200 ml.

2. Tris–HCl buffer (pH 7.2)

Mix 50 ml of tris(hydroxymethyl) methylamine (Tris) solution (24.2 g in 500 ml of water) and 18.3 ml of 1N HCl. Adjust the total volume to 100 ml with distilled water.

3. Glycine–HCl buffer (pH 2.4)

To 50 ml of a 0.2 M solution of glycine (15.01 g in 1000 ml of water) add 32.4 ml of 0.2 M HCl. Mix and adjust the total volume to 200 ml with distilled water.

4. Acetate buffer for linking of antigens to cyanogen bromide-activated Sephadex®

Add 41 ml 0.2 M acetic acid (11.55 ml/l) to 9 ml of 0.2 M sodium acetate (27.2 g/l of $C_2H_3O_4Na$. $3H_2O$), mix and adjust the final volume to 100 ml with distilled water.

5. Phosphate-buffered saline (PBS) (pH 7.2)

This contains 4.35 g of monobasic sodium phosphate ($NaH_2PO_4.2H_2O$), 10.15 g of dibasic sodium phosphate (Na_2HPO_4) and 9 g of NaCl per litre of distilled water; 0.1 g of sodium azide can be added if desired, although this must be avoided if the laboratory has lead or copper drain-pipes because of the risk of explosions.

GENERAL METHODS

Globulin precipitation

Add an equal volume of 36% sodium sulphate to the serum, drop by drop, whilst the mixture is being vigorously stirred. The reaction is carried out at room temperature and the precipitate which forms is separated by centrifugation at $2000\,g$ for 10 min at room temperature. The supernatant is discarded and the precipitate is dissolved in 0.15 M NaCl, using as small a volume as possible. After dissolution, the solution is dialysed against PBS (pH 7.2) for 24 h, with at least two changes of buffer.

Ammonium sulphate (saturated) can be used instead of sodium sulphate, but the reaction must then be carried out at 4 °C.

Freund's adjuvants

Freund's incomplete adjuvant

The antigen of interest is in aqueous solution (e.g. in saline) and is made up to 50% (v/v) in a Drakeol/Arlacel-A mixture (9 parts of Drakeol to 1 part of Arlacel-A). This complex is emulsified using a mechanical mixer or by pumping the fluid in and out of a 1-ml (tuberculin) syringe. The adjuvant should be periodically tested by dropping a small amount on to the surface of water in a beaker. If the droplet breaks up, further mixing is required until a discrete and complete 'spot' of adjuvant is obtained.

Freund's complete adjuvant

The procedure is as above, except that 1 mg of killed and dried *Mycobacterium tuberculosis* is added with the Drakeol. Care should be taken not to aerosolize this adjuvant if the investigator is hypersensitive to tuberculo-protein, otherwise a severe hypersensitivity reaction may result.

REAGENTS AND EQUIPMENT

Readers should note that the following list is not exhaustive and is not intended to be exclusive; it indicates only some sources which we have found helpful.

146

1. Antisera/immunoplates

Accurate Chemical & Scientific Corp.,
300 Shames Drive, Westbury, N.Y. 11590, USA.

Cappel Labs,
Cochranville, Pa. 19330, USA.

Hoechst Ltd.,
Hoechst House, Sailsbury Road, Hounslow, Middlesex TW4 6JH, UK.

Hyland Ltd (Diagnostics),
Caxton Way, Thetford, Norfolk IP24 3SE, UK.

Miles Labs. Inc.,
P.O. Box 2000, Elkhart, Ind. 46515, USA.

Nordic Immunological Labs.,
P.O. Box 3715, San Clemente, Calif. 92672, USA.

Pel-Freez,
P.O. Box 68, Rodgers, Ark. 72756, USA.

Sigma Chemicals Ltd.,
Fancy Road, Poole, Dorset BH17 7NH, UK.

2. Chemicals

Amersham Corp.,
2636 S. Clearbrook Drive, Arlington Heights, Ill. 60005, USA.

Amersham Ltd. (formerly The Radiochemical Centre Ltd.),
Amersham, Bucks., UK.

Atomic Energy Commission of Canada,
Tunneys Pasture, Ottawa, Ontario, Canada.

BDH Chemicals Ltd.,
Poole, Dorset, UK.

Calbiochem-Behring Corp.,
P.O. Box 12087, San Diego, Calif. 92112, USA.

Fisher Scientific Co.,
711 Forbes Ave., Pittsburgh, Pa. 15219, USA.

Kallestad Labs. Inc.,
1000 Lake Hazeltine Drive, Chaska, Minn. 55318, USA.
(suppliers of Kallestad IgE kits).

New England Nuclear,
549 Albany St., Boston, Mass., USA.

Pharmacia Fine Chemicals,
Piscataway, N.J. 08854, USA.

Pharmacia Ltd.,
Prince Regent Road, Hounslow, Middlesex TW3 1NE, UK.
(suppliers of RIST, Phadebas RAST® and Phadebas PRIST® kits—
Sepharose® Sephadex®, etc).
(NB. The above are registered trademarks of Pharmacia)

Sigma Chemical Co.,
P.O. Box 14508, St. Louis, Mo. 63178, USA.

Sigma Chemicals Ltd.
(see above).

3. Centrifuges

Beckman Instruments Inc.,
Spinco Div., 1117 California Ave.,
Palo Alto, Calif. 94304, USA.

Eppendorf Division,
Brinkmann Instruments Inc.,
Cantiague Rd., Westbury, N.Y.
11590, USA.

MSE Ltd.,
Gatwick Road, Crawley, Sussex,
RH10 2RP, UK

4. Automatic pipetting systems

Dynatech Labs. Inc.,
900 Slaters Lane, Alexandria, Va.
22314, USA.

Gilford Instruments Labs. Inc.,
132 Artino St., Oberlin, Ohio 44074,
USA.

Gilson Medical Electronics Inc.,
P.O. Box 27, 3000 W. Beltline,
Middleton, Wisc. 53562, USA.
(distributed by
Mandell Scientific Co. Ltd.,
395 Norman St.,
Ville St. Pierre,
Montreal, Quebec, Canada).

Hook and Turner Instruments Ltd.,
Vulcan Way, New Aldington,
Croydon, CR0 9UG, UK.

Micromedic Systems Div., Rohm &
Haas Co., Horsham, Pa. 19044, USA.

Scientific manufacturing Industries
Inc.,
800 University Avenue, Berkley,
Calif., USA.

Scientific Manufacturing Industries
Inc.,
1399 64th St., Emeryville, Calif.
94608, USA.

Geiger monitors

Mini Instruments Ltd.,
8 Station Industrial Estate,
Burnham-on-Crouch, Essex,
CM10 8RN, UK

Plastic spheres

Euromatic Ltd.,
Maycrete House, Boston Manor
Road, Brentford, Middlesex, UK

Precision Plastic Ball Co.
3000 N. Cicero Ave., Chicago, Illinois
60641

Blood packs and related products

Argyle,
Sherwood Medical, London Road,
County Oak, Crawley, West Sussex
RH10 2TL, UK

Baxter Division,
Travenol Laboratories Ltd.,
Thetford, Norfolk, UK

Biodec Inc.,
P.O. Box 3187, Cincinnati, Ohio,
45201, USA.

Cormed Inc.,
3 N. Main St., Middleport, N.Y.
14105, USA.

Dispensing pipettes

Cornwall Syringes,
Becton, Dickinson and Co.,
Rutherford, N.J., USA.

Eppendorf Division,
Brinkmann Instruments Inc. (see above).

Finn Pipettes,
Labsystems O.Y., Pulttitie 9. 00810,
Helsinki 81, Finland.

Gilson Medical Electronics Inc. (see above).

Fisher Scientific Co. (see above).

Scotlab Instrument Sales Ltd.,
Unit 15, Wildman Road Industrial Estate, Law, Carluke, Lanarkshire ML8 5E, UK.

5. Automatic washing systems

Dade (Division of American Hospital Supply),
Miami, Fla. 33152, USA.

Dynatech Labs. Inc. (see above).

Eppendorf Division, Brinkmann Instruments Inc. (see above).

Gilson Medical Electronics Inc. (see above).

Micromedic Systems Div., Rohm & Haas Co. (see above).

Ortho Pharmaceutical Ltd.,
Denmark House, Denmark Street, High Wycombe, Bucks., UK.

Sorvall Inc.,
Norwalk, Conn. 06856, USA
(British agents:
V. A. Howe and Co. Ltd.,
88 Peterborough Road, London, SW6, UK).

6. Gamma counters

Beckman Instruments Inc.,
Scientific Instruments Div., P.O. Box C-19600, Irvine, Calif. 92713, USA.

LKB Instruments Inc.,
12221 Parklawn Drive, Rockville, Ma. 20822, USA.

LKB Ltd.,
232 Addington Road, Selsdon, South Croydon CR2 BYD, UK.

Micromedic Systems Div., Rohm & Haas Co. (see above).

Nuclear Enterprises Ltd.,
Sighthill, Edinburgh,
EH11 4EY, UK.

Packard Instruments Ltd.,
13017 Church Road, Caversham,
Reading, Berks. RG4 7AA, UK.

GENERAL NOTES ON WORKING AREAS FOR RADIOIMMUNOASSAY

About half of the usual RIA procedure involves processing in which no radioactivity is involved. It is helpful to keep this part of the assay away from areas of the laboratory which are contaminated, or potentially contaminated, with radioisotopes. The isotope working area should be apart from other areas, i.e. in a separate room, which should have adequate warning notices for cleaners, etc., and should be equipped with fume cupboards, efficient ventilation, stainless-steel sinks and good working surfaces (see below for more detailed specifications). In addition, benches should be covered with a suitable absorptive material (e.g. Benchkote) which will trap spillages.

In the 'non-active' area one will require a centrifuge (we favour a machine which will achieve 3000 g, is refrigerated and will carry 100–300 75 × 12 mm plastic test-tubes), an orbital mixer, fixed-volume or variable-volume displacing pipettes (50–250 μl) and a magnetic stirrer base.

The same equipment is necessary for the 'active' part of the assay procedure. If the RIA is performed in two separate stages with different equipment in use at each stage, it will clearly be expensive in terms of capital expense. For this reason, it is often better to equip and use a radioisotope room which is used only for the assays and to take the same precautions for the 'non-active' and active parts of the assay, using a single set of equipment. All high-risk steps, such as dispensing or mixing isotope-labelled materials, should be performed in a fume cupboard.

Because large volumes of buffer are required, it is useful to have 20–30-litre containers with simple tap fitments, which are regularly filled with the appropriate solutions.

Gamma counters should be sited outside the radioisotope laboratory, in order to avoid contamination of the counting crystals which produces a permanently high background count. However, the area chosen to house the counter must be separate and must indicate clearly that it is a radioisotope area.

Radiolabelling of proteins must be carried out only in rigorously controlled areas and with well trained personnel, for the activities being handled are usually high. Ideally, a special suite for handling such high levels of isotopes should be available, although it is recognized that this is rarely possible. If it is not available, a fume cupboard with adequate precautions should suffice. The fume cupboard should ideally have a stainless-steel floor or be covered with a suitable absorbent material and it should be well extracted. If there is no stainless-steel base all operations should be performed in a large tray which can easily be decontaminated. Fig. 3.2 shows an isotope-labelling area in Ninewells Hospital, Dundee.

USE OF RADIOISOTOPES

These notes are based on the *Handbook of Radiological Protection*, published by Her Majesty's Stationery Office, London. The interested reader is advised to consult this publication.

A *radiological safety officer* should be appointed to over-see all radioisotope work. This person should have received adequate training and should have access to an experienced physicist for advice. He/she is responsible for general safety precautions and for keeping records of spillage, accidents, monitoring, stocks of isotopes and disposal of waste.

In the UK no person aged under 16 years (in the USA under 18 years) can work with radioactive substances and careful supervision is necessary for those aged 16–18 years. All workers should be correctly instructed on the hazards of working with isotopes.

The isotope working area should be set aside from other areas and clearly labelled. It should be carefully planned and have impermeable bench surfaces (e.g. Formica or vinyl) and sealed floors and surrounds. The bench surface should 'run' upwards on the wall surface for several inches so that the risk of splashes on to the wall is minimized. Two sinks, one for the disposal of radioactive waste and a separate one for hand-washing, will be required.

Instruments (Geiger monitors) should be available (suitable for the isotope in use) and should be used to monitor the working surfaces every day or several times a day. These instruments are not usually very sensitive and are designed to detect only gross contamination. A typical instrument is the Mini-monitor Type 5.40 scintillation meter with an X-ray probe Type 5.42 (Mini-Instruments Ltd.). Advice on the selection of a suitable instrument can be obtained from the National Radiological Protection Board, Harwell, Didcot, Oxon., UK.

Isotopes in storage should be clearly labelled, specifying the isotope, the name of the user and marked with warning tape. The isotope should be in leakproof containers and enclosed in a lead container or shielded by a wall of lead.

The disposal of radioactive waste must be carefully monitored (see below). In addition to the precautions noted above, it must be added that monitoring with a Geiger counter is an inaccurate method which detects only gross contamination of surfaces or equipment. It is therefore recommended that 'wipe tests' using alcohol-soaked swabs are also performed on surfaces, etc. The latter should be 'wiped' once a week and the swabs counted for radioactivity in a gamma counter. The results should be recorded, and a continuous record maintained.

Disposal of waste

Contaminated plastic equipment and glassware should be kept separate from non-contaminated materials. With some of these materials, e.g. plastic tubes, the radioactivity can be effectively washed out with several rinses, and provided that the residual activity is monitored with a Geiger counter before disposal it is safe to dispose of these items by incineration. However, when one is using glassware, it is expensive to discard and decontamination must be as efficient as possible. Most of the contamination will be due to radiolabelled protein which has non-specifically attached to the surface of the glass. Soaking in a strong detergent (e.g. Decon 20%; Decon Laboratories Ltd., Conway Street, Hove BN 3LY, UK) for 24–48 h will usually loosen this binding and the residual activity can be washed free. This is also a useful procedure with plastic equipment which retains a high activity after several rinses.

In National Health Service hospitals in the UK, the permitted levels of radioactive waste contamination for disposal without authorization are as follows:

Route	Limits
Sewerage	.10 mCi/month (public sewer)
	2 mCi/month (other sewer)
Solid waste..	.10 μCi/3 cu. ft. (no single item > 1 μCi)
Incineration	.10 μCi/batch (30 μCi/day)

Individual precautions

The individual worker should:
1. always wear a laboratory coat or gown and protective disposable gloves;
2. never pipette by mouth;
3. not make aerosols of isotopes or work with volatile isotopes in an open laboratory;
4. not drink, eat or smoke in an 'open' area;
5. prevent the spread of any spillage of isotope;
6. decontaminate all areas of spillage or ordinary contamination;
7. always wash hands thoroughly after working with radioactive substances even though protective gloves have been worn.

Maximum permitted radiation levels

In the UK, the maximum permitted contamination levels are:

Laboratory bench .. ..10^{-4} μCi/cm^2

Laboratory bench used exclusively for isotope work .. ..10^{-3} μCi/cm^2

Skin and clothing .. ..10^{-4} μCi/cm^2

The maximum permissible body burden of iodine-125 is 10 μCi. If this amount is present, it will be concentrated in the thyroid and can be easily demonstrated by monitoring the thyroid of the individual with a Geiger monitor at the neck. A suitable instrument can be obtained from Mini-Instruments Ltd., and it is strongly recommended that all workers are regularly monitored (1–2-week intervals), for this method detects technical mishandling in addition to defining maximum body burdens.

A SIMPLE BASIC COMPUTER PROGRAM FOR RIA OF ANTIBODY

The program shown in Fig. A.1 is provided for illustration of simple requirements. Other features may be found desirable by different workers and should

152

```
100 REM ************************************************************************
110 REM ***            SIMPLE RADIO-IMMUNE ASSAY PROGRAM.              ***
120 REM ***            BY W.J.HERBERT & V.S. MANDRANJAN.               ***
130 REM ************************************************************************
140 PRINT "ENTER NUMBER OF DOUBLING DILUTIONS OF THE STANDARD SERUM"
150 INPUT ND
160 N = ND
170 PRINT "WHAT IS THE FIRST DILUTION, E.G. 0.5 OR 0.25 ETC."
180 INPUT FD
190 PRINT
200 PRINT "-TO OMIT A READING FROM THE CALCULATION ENTER 0 INSTEAD OF COUNT-"
210 PRINT
220 FOR I = 1 TO ND
230 D = FD / (2^(I - 1))
240 PRINT "ENTER THE COUNT FOR"D"DILUTION"
250 INPUT C
260 IF C = 0 THEN GOTO 350
270 D = LOG(D)
280 C = LOG(C)
290 E = E + D
300 F = F + C
310 G = G + D^2
320 H = H + C^2
330 B = B + D*C
340 GOTO360
350 N = N - 1
360 NEXT I
370 J = (N*B - F*E) / (N*G - E^2)
380 K = (F - J*E) / N
390 E = J*(B - E*F / N)
400 H = H - F^2 / N
410 R = E / H
420 PRINT"CORRELATION COEFFICIENT ="SQR(R)
430 PRINT
440 PRINT"ENTER THE COUNT FOR THE TEST SERUM"
450 INPUT C
460 C = LOG(C)
470 PRINT"THIS CORRESPONDS TO DILUTION "EXP((C - K) / J)
480 PRINT
490 GOTO440
500 END
```

Figure A.1. BASIC computer program for RIA of antibody. $^\wedge$ = 'raise to power'

be added where necessary to the scheme shown. We are indebted to W. J. Herbert and J. S. Mandranjan of the University of Dundee for writing the program.

The program assumes that a doubling dilution series is used for the standard. Neat and 1-in-2 (0.5) dilutions can often be seen by inspection to be 'off' the regression (see Chapter 5) and should not then be used as entry data for the computer. The correlation coefficient calculated using the program should fall between 0.96 and 1 if the data are to be regarded as acceptable. If this is the case, the computer will then calculate 'equivalent dilutions' or units of antibody for each count entered for test sera.

The program contains no safeguards for operator errors, etc., and assumes that the variables will be zeroed before each run.

STANDARDIZATION OF RAST ASSAYS

As indicated in Chapter 6, the results of RAST assays for IgE antibody to allergens may be reported as a score or by comparison with dilutions of a standard serum.

With the score system:

  0 = antibody is undetectable
  1 = antibody is low
  2 = antibody is moderate
  3 = antibody is high
  4 = antibody is very high

With the dilution method:

  Dilution D = 0.35 Phadebas RAST units (PRU)/ml
  Dilution C = 0.7 Phadebas RAST units (PRU)/ml
  Dilution B = 3.5 Phadebas RAST units (PRU)/ml
  Dilution A = 17.5 Phadebas RAST units (PRU)/ml

INDEX

156